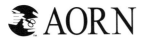 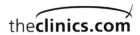

PERIOPERATIVE NURSING CLINICS

Bariatric Surgery

Brenda S. Gregory Crum, RN, MSN, CNOR
Guest Editor

Patricia C. Seifert, RN, MSN, CNOR, CRNFA, FAAN
Consulting Editor

March 2006 • Volume 1 • Number 1

SAUNDERS

An Imprint of Elsevier, Inc.
PHILADELPHIA   LONDON   TORONTO   MONTREAL   SYDNEY   TOKYO

W.B. SAUNDERS COMPANY

A Division of Elsevier Inc.

Elsevier Inc. • 1600 John F. Kennedy Boulevard • Suite 1800 • Philadelphia, Pennsylvania 19103-2899

http://www.periopnursing.theclinics.com

PERIOPERATIVE NURSING CLINICS   Volume 1, Number 1
March 2006   ISSN 1556-7931
Editor: Maria Lorusso   ISBN 1-4160-3566-4

The ideas and opinions expressed in *Perioperative Nursing Clinics* do not necessarily reflect those of the Publisher. The Publisher does not assume any responsibility for any injury and/or damage to persons or property arising out of or related to any use of the material contained in this periodical. The reader is advised to check the appropriate medical literature and the product information currently provided by the manufacturer of each drug to be administered to verify the dosage, the method and duration of administration, or contraindications. It is the responsibility of the treating physician or other health care professional, relying on independent experience and knowledge of the patient, to determine drug dosages and the best treatment for the patient. Mention of any product in this issue should not be construed as endorsement by the contributors, editors, or the Publisher of the product or manufacturers' claims.

The Perioperative Nursing Clinics (ISSN 1556-7931) is published quarterly by W.B. Saunders, 360 Park Avenue South, New York, NY 10010-1710. Months of publication are March, June, September, and December. Business and Editorial Offices: 1600 John F. Kennedy Boulevard, Suite 1800, Philadelphia, PA 19103-2899. Accounting and Circulation Offices: 6277 Sea Harbor Drive, Orlando, FL 32887-4800. Periodicals postage paid at New York, NY and additional mailing offices. Subscription prices are $99.00 per year (US individuals), $160.00 per year (US institutions), $50.00 per year (US students), $120.00 per year (Canadian and foreign individuals), $180.00 per year (Canadian and foreign institutions), and $50.00 per year (Canadian and foreign students). Foreign air speed delivery is included in all Clinics subscription prices. All prices are subject to change without notice. **POSTMASTER:** Send address changes to *The Perioperative Nursing Clinics*, Elsevier Periodicals Customer Service, 6277 Sea Harbor Drive, Orlando, FL 32887-4800. Customer Service: 1-800-654-2452 (US). From outside of the US, call 1-407-345-4000.

Perioperative Nursing Clinics is covered in *Index Medicus, Current Contents/Clinical Medicine, EMBASE/ Excerpta Medica, Science Citation Index, and ISI/BIOMED.*

Printed in the United States of America.

CONSULTING EDITOR

PATRICIA C. SEIFERT, RN, MSN, CNOR, CRNFA, FAAN, Education Coordinator, Cardiovascular Operating Room, Inova Heart and Vascular Institute, Falls Church, Virginia

GUEST EDITOR

BRENDA S. GREGORY CRUM, RN, MSN, CNOR, Safety Ambassador, Sandel Medical Industries LLC, Chatsworth, California

CONTRIBUTORS

CHERI ACKERT-BURR, RN, MSN, CNOR, Clinical Consultant, US Surgical, Norwalk, Connecticut

LORRAINE J. BUTLER, RN, BSN, MSA, CNOR, Administrative Director, Methodist Hospital, Clarian Health Partners, Indianapolis, Indiana

ROBIN CHARD, MSN, RN, CNOR, PhD candidate, Clinical Assistant Professor of Nursing, Florida International University School of Nursing, Miami, Florida

BRENDA S. GREGORY CRUM, RN, MSN, CNOR, Safety Ambassador, Sandel Medical Industries LLC, Chatsworth, California

MALENE K. INGRAM, MD, Advanced Laparoscopic Gastrointestinal and Bariatric Surgery Fellow, Interdisciplinary Obesity Treatment Group, Department of Surgery, University of South Florida Health Sciences Center, Tampa General Hospital, Tampa, Florida

MICHEL M. MURR, MD, FACS, Director of Bariatric Surgery, Associate Professor of Surgery, Department of Surgery, University of South Florida Health Sciences Center, Tampa General Hospital, Tampa, Florida

DENISE O'BRIEN, MSN, APRN,BC, FAAN, Clinical Nurse Specialist, Department of Operating Rooms/PACU, University of Michigan Hospitals and Health Centers, Ann Arbor, Michigan

WILLIAM C. PALAZZOLO, MS, PA-C, Physician Assistant, University of Michigan Hospital General Surgery Clinic Support; and Program Director, Bariatric Surgery, University of Michigan Hospitals and Health Centers, Ann Arbor, Michigan

LYNN RANDALL, RN, BSN, MBA-HCM, Clinical Consultant, US Surgical, Norwalk, Connecticut

RITA C. SCHEIDT, RNC, BSN, Staff Educator, Department of Continuing Education and Staff Development, MedCentral Health System, Mansfield, Ohio

CONTENTS

> Obesity is an epidemic with poorly understood root causes. The medical and economic burden of obesity far exceeds many other epidemics in recent history. Dietary and behavior modification and pharmaceutical interventions result in modest and short-lived weight loss. Bariatric surgery is the only current treatment that results in significant, durable, and sustainable weight loss that is associated with resolution of comorbidities, improvement in quality of life, and significant reduction in health care cost savings. This article reviews current concepts in treatment with emphasis on perioperative care of bariatric patients.

> With the rising trend of obesity, the number of bariatric surgeries has risen significantly as an alternative to managing this prevalent condition. This review of the literature focuses on the comorbid factors, patient selection, and health care costs associated with obesity and bariatric surgery.

> Patients who choose bariatric surgery have faced not only the health consequences associated with obesity but have endured stigma and shame. Health care providers must recognize that bias and prejudice toward the obese leads to stereotyping and ultimately the devaluation and marginalization of this population. Health care providers are not immune; they manifest the same bias resident in western culture. Professionals in health care must increase awareness of their own perceptions and attitudes. This article

contributes to the eradication of this prejudice. A deeper sense of empathy leads to improved patient outcomes and contributes to health promotion, not only for the bariatric surgery patient, but also for every patient who struggles with weight.

for some, for others it has the potential for failure. Clinicians serve patients best by a proactive commitment, by joining forces with them in their quest for the pivotal answer. Engaging in candid dialog and sharing their journey, by telling the truth without sensationalizing the facts, make truth telling an adjunct to bariatric care.

The bariatric population offers unique challenges and requires health care providers to understand potential problems and promote safe practices. This article reviews high-risk considerations for bariatric care including education, resource allocation, airway and medication management, positioning, and prevention of postoperative complications. The environmental needs, resource needs, and problem-prone interventions that must be considered when planning and caring for these patients are discussed.

FORTHCOMING ISSUES

ELSEVIER
SAUNDERS

Perioperative Nursing Clinics 1 (2006) ix

PERIOPERATIVE
NURSING
CLINICS

Foreword

Bariatric Surgery: A Multifaceted Challenge

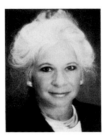

Patricia C. Seifert, RN, MSN, CNOR, CRNFA, FAAN
Consulting Editor

Welcome to the first issue of the *Perioperative Nursing Clinics*, a quarterly periodical in which each issue focuses on a single clinical topic. This premier issue on bariatric surgery illustrates the complexity of many clinical topics. In addition to clinical considerations, the obesity epidemic that has fueled the dramatic growth of bariatric surgery is associated with other relevant subjects that are addressed in this issue: comorbidities, prejudice and bias, ethical aspects, quality of life, patient and staff education, cost and business aspects, safety, and current research on the subject. Future issues focusing on vascular surgery, evidence-based practice, and endoscopic surgery, for example, will include a similar array of articles addressing educational, financial, research, qualitative, and technologic facets of the topic.

Another focus of the *Perioperative Nursing Clinics* is to highlight relevant standards, recommended practices, and guidelines from the Association of periOperative Registered Nurses (AORN) as well as other authoritative sources. The articles in the present issue include references to guidelines and recommendations from AORN, the American Society for Bariatric Surgery, Centers for Disease Control and Prevention, the Agency for Health Care Research and Quality, and the National Institute of Diabetes and Digestive and Kidney Diseases.

Guest editors and authors are selected on the basis of their expertise. In this issue, Brenda S. Gregory Crum, RN, MSN, CNOR, has assembled a multidisciplinary panel of experts who provide information and insights into the complex issues affecting patients undergoing bariatric surgery. In today's surgical environment, nurses, physicians, and other members of the health care team work together to affect patient outcomes; the *Perioperative Nursing Clinics* reflects the importance of including input from all members of the surgical team.

Looking at select perioperative issues from a variety of perspectives is an important benefit of the *Perioperative Nursing Clinics*. We look forward to presenting up-to-date information that will be useful in your practice. This issue is an excellent introduction to a complex topic, and Ms. Crum and her coauthors have set a high mark. We look forward to serving your needs with future issues.

Patricia C. Seifert, RN, MSN,
CNOR, CRNFA, FAAN
Cardiovascular Operating Room
Inova Heart and Vascular Institute
3300 Gallows Road
Falls Church, VA 22042, USA

E-mail address: patricia.seifert@inova.com

1556-7931/06/$ - see front matter © 2006 Elsevier Inc. All rights reserved.
doi:10.1016/j.cpen.2006.01.003

ELSEVIER
SAUNDERS

Perioperative Nursing Clinics 1 (2006) xi–xii

PERIOPERATIVE
NURSING
CLINICS

Preface

Treatment or Prevention: Eliminating Obesity

The focus on bariatric surgery and obesity in this issue of the *Perioperative Nursing Clinics* emphasizes the special program and patient care needs of the obese population to improve outcomes. Authors provide a wealth of information related to the bariatric population. Articles in this issue describe the research related to comorbid conditions, treatment options, education needs of the healthcare team, and care in the Intensive Care Unit. The prejudice, bias, and stigma associated with obesity, as well as the power of interpretation of facts, are addressed to help us understand how opinions are formed. In addition, articles summarize the business case for a bariatric program and safety issues when caring for this population. The subspecialty of bariatrics has evolved because of an obvious obesity epidemic. The knowledge needed to care for this population has increased awareness and knowledge about heart disease, stroke, cancer, and diabetes—all high-risk diseases associated with obesity. The circle of influence extends to the care of many other patients in all specialties undergoing surgical procedures. Although the emphasis for health care providers is treatment and care of everyone who enters our facilities, our understanding of adverse lifestyle choices and habits is invaluable to address the obesity epidemic.

Community movement for prevention

The program *Activate America: Pioneering Healthier Communities* was started in July 2004 by the United States YMCA because of overwhelming statistics associated with obesity and the obvious effect within communities. Attention-getting data from the Centers for Disease Control and Prevention that is related to this prevalent, costly, and preventive epidemic include:

- Nearly 59 million adults are obese. Moreover, the epidemic is not limited to adults: the percentage of young people who are overweight has more than doubled in the last 20 years.
- Chronic diseases such as heart disease, cancer, and diabetes are leading causes of disability and death in the United States.
- 125 million Americans live with one or more chronic diseases, and 70% of the nation's total medical care costs go toward treating individuals who have these conditions.
- More than 1.7 million Americans die of chronic diseases each year, accounting for 70% of all deaths in the United States.
- If current trends continue, deaths attributed to poor diet and lack of physical activity may soon surpass smoking-attributable deaths.
- Despite the proven benefits of physical activity, more than 50% of American adults do not get enough physical activity to provide health benefits: 26% are not active at all in their leisure time.
- 33% of all deaths in the United States (about 800,000 deaths each year) can be attributed to a lack of physical activity and poor eating habits [1].

Envisioning a need for a social response, the YMCA selected 14 communities to focus on replicating healthy community models that are proven to work. The YMCA worked with national experts from organizations such as the Robert Wood Johnson Foundation, the Centers for Disease Control and Prevention, the US Department of Health and Human Services, and others to determine criteria for an active program. Community leaders were invited to join their team to help improve lifestyles for their citizens.

In July 2004, two Chief Executive Officers of the YMCA were invited to testify during the US Senate Appropriations Subcommittee hearing on "Healthy Communities and Wellness" with Secretary Tommy Thompson of the US Department

doi:10.1016/j.cpen.2006.01.002

of Health and Human Services. In September 2004, the 14 community teams went to Washington, DC, for a conference where they developed working plans based on evidence-based, model practices in public policy and programs. These teams' purpose is to meet the needs of all Americans for healthier and more life-enhancing ways to live and advance common strategies to remove barriers and increase support for healthy living for individuals and families.

Making the choice for prevention

As individuals, we make choices for ourselves and our families. As health care providers, we have a better understanding of the repercussions of bad decisions and see the results of those decisions everyday. As Americans, we are choosing to support an epidemic if we ignore the facts. A healthier future begins at home with attention to unhealthy lifestyles including nutrition and physical activity levels and a commitment to understand and address the problem.

Expanding the initiative by raising awareness and participating in a community-wide movement can help reverse trends and possibly make bariatric care nonexistent. The Activate America program is a partnership model to address what the YMCA claims is a "big, hairy, audacious goal" that can change the way Americans live. In 2005, an additional 20 communities joined forces to mirror the experiences of the original 14 pioneers. As registered nurses, practicing the best treatment regimens is crucial. As individuals and groups, registered nurses have the resources to take on the role of prevention to improve physical, social, emotional, and spiritual health that is a basis for the greater need of a healthier society. Let's benefit from the knowledge we have gleaned to practice the best care and treatment while necessary—but shift our priorities to prevention to wipe out this prevalent obesity epidemic.

Brenda S. Gregory Crum, RN, MSN, CNOR
11105 Castleberry Road
Odessa, FL 34655, USA

E-mail address: bsgd@aol.com

Reference

[1] YMCA. YMCA Activate America. Available at: http://www.ymca.net/activateamerica/. Accessed January 11, 2006.

**ELSEVIER
SAUNDERS**

Perioperative Nursing Clinics 1 (2006) 1–7

PERIOPERATIVE
NURSING
CLINICS

Overview of the Treatment of Obesity

Malene K. Ingram, MD, Michel M. Murr, MD, FACS*

*Department of Surgery, University of South Florida Health Sciences Center, Tampa General Hospital,
2 Columbia Drive, Tampa, FL 33601, USA*

Obesity is a worldwide epidemic. Approximately 63 million Americans are classified as obese, and 55% of adults aged 20 and older are overweight or obese [1]. The classification of overweight and obese (Table 1) is based on determination of body mass index (BMI), which is calculated by dividing the weight (kilograms) by the square of height (meters) [2]. The term "morbid obesity" has been largely replaced by clinically significant obesity or severe obesity. It is estimated that at least 3% of the United States population or approximately 5 million people [1] meet the weight criteria for bariatric surgery (BMI ≥ 40 or ≥ 35 kg/m^2 with severe comorbidities) [3].

Nonoperative treatment

Clinical guidelines from the evidence-based National Heart, Lung and Blood Institute on treatment of overweight and obesity in adults, weight loss, and maintenance therapy recommend a combination of low-calorie diets, exercise, and behavioral therapy as first-line treatment [4]. Specifically, behavioral therapy should incorporate strategies to promote changes in diet, eating habits, and exercise through acquisition of motivation and support [5]. The 2004 American Society for Bariatric Surgery consensus conference found that high-intensity well-designed behavioral treatment using diet and exercise counseling could achieve a weight loss of approximately 8% to 10% of baseline weight [5].

Very low calorie (< 800 kcal/d) diets replace usual food intake with enriched protein meals and micronutrients. These diets produce substantial weight losses within 12 to 24 weeks compared with low-calorie diets (< 1600 kcal/d); however, the long-term weight loss is comparable with low-calorie diets [5]. Additionally, weight loss is faster with low-carbohydrate diets compared with low-fat diets but the long-term (> 6 months) weight loss is similar [6].

Pharmacotherapy is used as an adjunct to diet and exercise in patients with a BMI > 30 or those with a BMI > 27 and weight-related comorbidities. The two Food and Drug Administration approved drugs (sibutramine, a serotonin-epinephrine reuptake inhibitor that acts as an appetite suppressant; and orlistat, a competitive intestinal lipase inhibitor that blocks the absorption of dietary fats) induce modest weight loss (5–10 kg). Chronic medication use and behavioral therapy are needed to sustain long-term weight loss [5].

Operative treatment

Bariatric surgery is the most effective modality for substantial and durable weight loss. The American Society for Bariatric Surgery estimates that 140,000 weight-loss procedures have been undertaken in 2004. Surgically induced weight loss is associated with improvement in obesity-related comorbidities including diabetes, hypertension, obstructive sleep apnea (OSA), gastroesophageal reflux disease, and reduction in use of medications and health care expenditure [7,8]. Additionally, there is improved quality of life in patients with clinically significant obesity who undergo bariatric surgery.

Preoperative interdisciplinary team evaluation

Before any operative intervention, a comprehensive evaluation by an interdisciplinary team is

---

* Corresponding author.
E-mail address: mmurr@hsc.usf.edu (M.M. Murr).

doi:10.1016/j.cpen.2005.12.007

Table 1
Classification of obesity

Obesity class	BMI (kg/m^2)
Underweight	<18.5
Normal	18.5–24.9
Overweight	25.0–29.9
Mild obesity I	30.0–34.9
Moderate obesity II	35.0–39.9
Severe obesity III	≥ 40.0

Table 2
Comorbidities of obesity

Neurologic	Pseudotumor cerebri
Circulatory	Hypertension
	Cardiomyopathy
	Venous stasis disease
	Pulmonary hypertension
	Deep venous thrombosis
Pulmonary	Obstructive sleep apnea
	Obesity hypoventilation syndrome
Gastrointestinal	Gastroesophageal reflux disease
	Cholelithiasis
	Nonalcoholic steatotic hepatitis
Genitourinary or gynecologic	Stress urinary incontinence
	Polycystic ovary syndrome
Musculoskeletal	Mechanical arthropathy
Metabolic	Diabetes mellitus
	Hyperlipidemia
	Hypercholesterolemia
	Syndrome X
Psychiatric	Depression
	Binge eating disorder
	Somatization disorder
	Body dysmorphic disorders

important to screen and treat medical comorbidities and to establish behavior modification and dietary counseling. Obesity is an independent risk factor for postoperative morbidity and mortality. Specifically, male gender, age greater than 55 years, BMI >50 kg/m^2, and hypertension are predictive of a complicated postoperative course [9,10].

The authors' interdisciplinary team includes a bariatric surgeon, a bariatrician, a bariatric nutritionist, and a psychologist. The bariatric surgeon should devote a good portion of his or her surgical practice toward caring for obese patients, directing and coordinating the interdisciplinary team, and independently assessing the adequacy of the preoperative evaluation.

The bariatrician can be a family practitioner or an internist who is specifically attuned to the needs of obese patients. The bariatrician evaluates, identifies, and directs treatment of obesity-related conditions (Table 2), such as control of hypertension, diabetes mellitus, and dyslipidemia. This also includes recognition and evaluation of previous myocardial infarction or ischemia, cardiomyopathy, and dysrhythmias. The evaluation includes ECG, echocardiogram, dobutamine stress test or nuclear myocardial scintigraphy, cardiac catheterization, and sleep study as needed. The bariatrician ensures that the proper evaluation and treatment of comorbidities occurs before and after surgery, and adjusts medications as the patient's comorbidities resolve with weight loss.

The bariatric nutritionist has the role of identifying eating preferences and any nutritional deficiencies secondary to previous weight loss attempts. The nutritionist works with the patient after the operative intervention in developing a diet plan and assisting the patient with understanding the dietary ramifications of bariatric surgery (ie, diet restriction, dumping syndrome, and life-long vitamin and mineral supplementation).

A bariatric mental health advisor who can be a psychiatrist or a psychologist is an essential member of the interdisciplinary team because of the high prevalence rates of depression, anxiety, binge eating, body dysmorphic disorders, and somatization in bariatric patients [11,12]. Because psychologic characteristics, personality, and eating behavior may affect treatment outcomes, the bariatric psychologist thoroughly evaluates and identifies factors that may affect prognosis [11,12] and develops individual treatment plans.

Additionally, preoperative evaluation may include further consultations with other specialists for obesity-related comorbidities, such as OSA and hypercoagulability. More than 60% of bariatric patients suffer from OSA, and many do not have the typical symptoms of heavy snoring, witnessed apnea, fatigue, and excess daytime sleepiness. The authors routinely screen patients with the Epworth Sleepiness Scale [13,14] and refer them to a sleep laboratory for formal sleep study if they score >6. Additionally, they require patients with OSA to use their continuous positive airway pressure and bilevel positive airway pressure (BiPAP) machines for at least 4 weeks preoperatively for alveolar recruitment and to reverse alveolar hypoventilation [15].

Most importantly, perioperative thromboprophylaxis with low-molecular-weight heparin is mandatory and extended prophylaxis (after discharge from hospital) is continued for 2 weeks in patients with BMI >60, immobility, or previous history of thromboembolic events. Additionally, the authors recommend prophylactic preoperative placement of an inferior vena cava filter in patients with pulmonary embolism, prior deep venous thrombosis, lower-extremity venous stasis, or known hypercoagulable states [16]. Furthermore, the authors require patients to stop smoking to minimize the likelihood of thromboembolic events [17].

An integral part of preoperative evaluation and education is to engage prospective patients in peer counseling through biweekly support groups and educational seminars.

Bariatric procedures

The basic concepts of bariatric surgery have been gastric restriction or malabsorption [18]. The first malabsorptive procedure, done in the 1950s, was the jejunocolic bypass, which was complicated by severe diarrhea. This led to a modification of the procedure to a jejuno-ileal bypass that involved bypassing a large portion of the small bowel (Fig. 1A). This procedure is no longer undertaken because of the severe metabolic sequelae of acute hepatic failure, cirrhosis, oxalate kidney stones, and oxalate-induced nephropathy, along with protein-calorie, vitamin, and mineral nutritional deficiencies.

Other weight loss procedures that are no longer done because of poor weight loss include various gastroplasties (stomach stapling), which involve partitioning of the stomach with communication to the rest of the stomach by a narrow channel or stoma. The most notable of the gastroplasties is the vertical banded gastroplasty, which was common in 1980 and is no longer done. This restrictive procedure involved stapling of the stomach followed by placement of a silicone or polypropylene mesh, which bands or rings the channel or stoma externally (see Fig. 1B). Long-term weight loss is insufficient because of staple line breakdown and maladaptive eating behavior (ie, ice cream, sodas, and so forth).

Other unsuccessful procedures include the loop gastric bypass, which was complicated by severe bile reflux esophagitis, and the partial biliopancreatic diversion (see Fig. 1C), which is associated with a high incidence of protein-calorie malnutrition and severe steatorrhea.

Roux-en-Y gastric bypass

Currently the gold standard, the Roux-en-Y gastric bypass (RYGB) combines restrictive and maldigestive properties. A small pouch (<30 mL) is separated from the distal stomach by staples and connected to the proximal jejunum (see Fig. 1D). Thereby, ingested food bypasses the stomach, duodenum, and the proximal jejunum. Laparoscopic RYGB has become the procedure of choice because of reduction in wound complications, pain, length of hospital stay, and earlier return to daily activities.

Weight loss generally has been >60% of the excess body weight at 2 years with gradual mean weight gain such that the mean percent weight loss remains excellent at >50% excess body weight (Table 3) at 5- and 10-years postoperatively [7]. Reduction or resolution of obesity-related comorbidities is reported to be 93% for gastroesophageal reflux disease, 86% for diabetes mellitus, 86% for OSA, 78% for hypertension, 70% for hyperlipidemia, and 50% for mechanical arthropathy (Table 4) [8,19].

Overall complications are <10% and overall mortality is 1% to 2% (see Table 3) [8]. Early complications (range, 1%–2%) are anastomotic leak, sepsis, pulmonary embolism, deep venous thrombosis, bleeding, myocardial infarction, and stroke [7]; wound infection is more common in open versus laparoscopic procedures (15% versus 2%). Late complications include incisional hernia, anastomotic stricture, ulcers, gastrointestinal bleeding, and small bowel obstruction (Table 5). Nutritional deficiencies of iron, calcium, or vitamin B_{12} cause anemia, fatigue, osteoporosis, and neuropathies, and are best avoided by routine daily intake of these supplements.

Laparoscopic adjustable gastric banding

This purely restrictive procedure was first introduced in Europe in the 1990s as an alternative to the vertical banded gastroplasty and RYGB. A silicone band is placed around the cardia of the stomach, and its inner diameter is adjusted by a subcutaneous implanted reservoir (see Fig. 1E). Band adjustments are performed in the office until steady weight loss of 1 to 2 pounds per week is achieved. There is less of a risk of complications and malnutrition compared with the other restrictive and malabsorptive procedures; however, weight loss is slower and may plateau at 18 to 24 months (see Table 3). Complications include gastric prolapse, band slippage, band malposition, band erosion, port migration, port infection, tubing leak, and port leak (see Table 5), all of which require surgical intervention to repair.

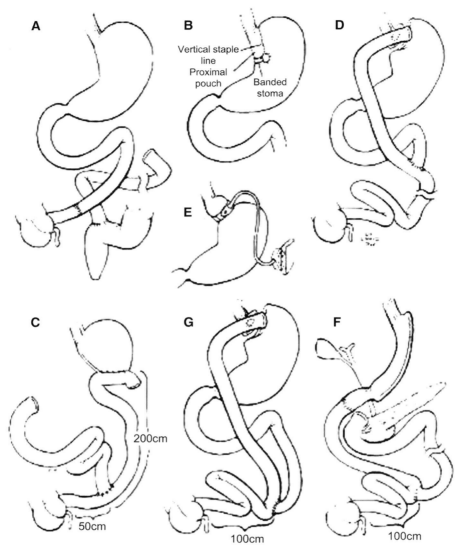

Fig. 1. Schematic drawings of bariatric procedures. (*A*) Jejuno-ileal bypass. (*B*) Vertical banded gastroplasty; the stoma is banded by a polypropylene mesh or polymeric silicone ring. (*C*) Malabsorptive: partial pancreaticobiliary bypass involves a partial gastrectomy and a gastroileostomy. (*D*) Roux-en-Y gastric bypass. (*E*) Adjustable gastric banding; the band is connected to a reservoir place in the subcutaneous tissue. (*F*) Biliopancreatic bypass with duodenal switch. (*G*) Very long Roux-en-Y gastric bypass shortens the common channel to 100 cm. *C*, *F*, and *G* are used in superobese patients and infrequently undertaken in North America. (*From* Balsiger BM, Murr MM, Poggio JL, et al. Bariatric surgery: surgery for weight control in patients with morbid obesity. Med Clin North Am 2000;84:482; with permission.)

Weight loss data beyond 4 years from United States centers is scant.

Duodenal switch with biliopancreatic diversion

This procedure involves tubularizing the stomach and anastomosing the transected duodenum to the ileum (see Fig. 1F). As with RYGB, ingested food bypasses the duodenum and proximal jejunum. Weight loss is being reported as slightly better than the RYGB (see Table 3). Complications are similar to the RYGB (see Table 5); however, bile salt wasting, bile salt–induced secretory diarrhea, and depletion of total body bile salt

Table 3
Mean weight loss and mortality of various bariatric procedures

Procedure	Excess weight loss (%)	Mortality (%)
Gastric banding	41	0.1
Gastric bypass	62	0.5
Duodenal switch	70	1.1

pool leading to fat malabsorption and fat-soluble vitamin deficiencies can occur [1]. Long-term outcomes data are needed to evaluate fully this procedure.

Postoperative care

The postoperative care of the bariatric surgery patient requires close monitoring of cardiac and respiratory status. The most common unexpected cause of death in the morbidly obese following surgery is pulmonary embolism, which can be prevented by early ambulation and thromboprophylaxis. In the authors' series, age >50 years, history of smoking, history of deep venous thrombosis or pulmonary embolism, and anastomotic leaks were predictive of pulmonary embolism [15]. Clinically, patients present with tachycardia, dyspnea, pleuritic chest pain, hemoptysis, and hypoxemia.

Anastomotic leak is a dreaded complication because of its increased mortality. It occurs in 1% to 3% of RYGB [20], and the earliest sign is persistent tachycardia, abdominal pain not relieved by medication, and fever. Hypotension and oliguria are late and ominous findings [20]. Abdominal examinations are not reliable; upper gastrointestinal and CT scans may miss a leak in 50% of cases. A high index of suspicion should be maintained, and operative evaluation may be undertaken to determine the presence of a leak [3]. Failure to diagnose and treat an anastomotic leak most often

Table 4
Resolution of comorbidities after surgically induced weight loss

Comorbidity	Improved or resolved (%)
Gastroesophageal reflux disease	93
Diabetes	86
Obstructive sleep apnea	86
Hypertension	78
Hyperlipidemia	70
Mechanical arthropathy	50

leads to severe sepsis, multiple organ failure, and death [20].

Respiratory failure is another cause of early mortality, especially in patients with OSA. Continuous positive airway pressure should be instituted immediately in the recovery room in patients' with OSA; early and pre-emptive endotracheal intubation should be undertaken at the earliest sign of respiratory insufficiency in those patients with difficult airways.

Wound infection should be treated aggressively with antibiotics and open packing. The authors avoid opening the full length of the abdominal incision because of the inevitable subsequent wide gaping of wound edges. Treatment of these wounds has been facilitated by the use of suction pumps.

Vomiting and intolerance to liquids after surgery is abnormal and may indicate the development of stomal stenosis, bleeding, or bowel obstruction. Stomal stenosis, or narrowing of the gastrojejunostomy [20], requires endoscopic dilation. Small bowel obstruction in the immediate postoperative period is uncommon; 50% of patients who develop small bowel obstruction in the immediate postoperative period may require operative treatment for internal hernia and trocar site hernias.

Hematemesis is abnormal and may indicate the presence of anastomotic bleeding or marginal ulcers. Anastomotic ulcers are usually associated with nonsteroidal anti-inflammatory drug use. Patients may present with pain, hematemesis, melena, and orthostatic hypotension. Treatment includes acid suppression, endoscopic evaluation, and blood transfusion if bleeding is massive.

Long-term sequelae

Other complications that may develop in the long term (see Table 5) include symptomatic cholelithiasis, dumping syndrome, persistent vomiting, and nutritional deficiencies. Approximately, 30% to 50% of bariatric patients develop symptomatic cholelithiasis within 1 year of surgery secondary to rapid weight loss [7]. This can be prevented by concomitant cholecystectomy or treatment with bile salt therapy; however, the latter is expensive and has poor patient compliance.

Dumping syndrome results from the rapid movement of undigested carbohydrates into the small intestine, causing symptoms of diarrhea, nausea, hypotension, tachycardia, and dizziness

Table 5
Complications of bariatric surgery

Surgery	Early	Late
Roux-en-Y gastric bypass	Pulmonary embolus	Anastomotic stricture
	Anastomotic leak	Marginal ulcer
	Deep venous thrombosis	Gastrointestinal bleeding
	Gastrointestinal bleeding	Dumping syndrome
	Wound infection	Anemia
	Enterocutaneous fistula	Neuropathy-B_{12} deficiency
	Small bowel obstruction	Dermatitis
	Sepsis	Hair loss
	Respiratory failure	Weight gain
		Incisional hernia
		Small bowel obstruction
		Osteoporosis
		Malnutrition
Duodenal switch	Similar to Roux-en-Y gastric bypass	Bile salt wasting
		Diarrhea-secretory
		Malabsorption
		Vitamin deficiency
		Dermatitis
Laparoscopic adjustable gastric band	Gastric prolapse	Band erosion
	Band slippage	Port migration
	Band malposition	Port infection
	Gastric occlusion	Disconnection of port tubing
	Esophageal dilation	Malnutrition

[20]. Dumping is a self-limited event related to the ingestion of carbohydrates and usually resolves in 1 to 2 hours. Prevention is through diet modification and exclusion of high-carbohydrate foods.

Long-term nutritional deficiencies may be prevented by daily supplements including multivitamins, 1200 mg of calcium citrate, and monthly injections of 1000 µg vitamin B_{12}. Nevertheless, isolated deficiencies in iron, folate, and B_{12} levels occur in up to 40% of patients but clinically significant anemias are much less common (<5%) and are more frequent in menstruating women [21].

Special considerations

Care of the obese patients necessitates major changes in providers' attitude and approaches. Obesity-friendly furniture and hospital environment including operating room beds, stretchers, wheel chairs, x-ray tables, CT scanners, toilet seats, and beds have to be changed to meet certain weight criteria. More importantly, sensitivity training for all providers is essential for success of treatment and patient satisfaction.

Summary

Bariatric surgery is safe and provides durable and sustainable weight loss, amelioration of obesity-related comorbidities, and health care savings. Allied health personnel play a vital role in the care of obese patients and provide early recognition and intervention of complications and untoward events. Further research on patient safety in this changing care environment is warranted.

References

[1] Brechner RJ, Farris C, Harrison S, et al. A graded, evidence-based summary of evidence for bariatric surgery. Surgery of Obesity and Related Diseases 2005;1:430–1.

[2] Oria HE, Carrasquilla C, Cunningham P, et al. Guidelines for weight calculations and follow-up in bariatric surgery. Surgery of Obesity and Related Diseases 2005;1:67–8.

[3] Nelson LG, Murr M. Operative treatment of clinically significant obesity. Board review series. Hospital Physician 2005;8:2–12.

[4] National Institutes of Health. Clinical guidelines on the identification, evaluation, and treatment of overweight and obesity in adults: the evidence report. Obes Res 1998;6:51S–209.

[5] Kushner R. Diets, drugs, exercise, and behavioral modification: where these work and where they do

not. Surgery of Obesity and Related Diseases 2005;1:
120–2.

[6] Foster GD, Wyatt HR, Hill JO, et al. A randomized
trial of a low-carbohydrate diet for obesity. N Engl J
Med 2003;348:2082–90.

[7] Kral JG, Christou NV, Flum DR, et al. Medicare
and bariatric surgery. Surgery of Obesity and Related Diseases 2005;1:35–63.

[8] Buchwald H, Avidor Y, Braunwald E, et al. Bariatric surgery: a systematic review and meta-analysis.
JAMA 2004;292:1724–37.

[9] Livingston EH, Huerta S, Arthur D, et al. Male gender is a predictor of morbidity and age a predictor of
mortality for patients undergoing gastric bypass surgery. Ann Surg 2002;236:576–82.

[10] Gonzalez R, Bowers SP, Venkatesh KR, et al. Preoperative factors predictive of complicated postoperative management after Roux-en-Y gastric
bypass for morbid obesity. Surg Endosc 2003;17:
1900–4.

[11] Rosik CH. Psychiatric symptoms among prospective bariatric surgery patients: rates of prevalence
and their relation to social desirability, pursuit of
surgery, and follow-up attendance. Obes Surg 2005;
15:677–83.

[12] van Hout GC, van Oudheusden I, van Heck GL.
Psychological profile of the morbidly obese. Obes
Surg 2004;14:579–88.

[13] Rasheid S, Banasiak M, Gallagher S, et al. Gastric
bypass is an effective treatment for obstructive sleep

apnea in patients with clinically significant obesity.
Obes Surg 2003;13:58–61.

[14] Serafini FM, Anderson WM, Rosemurgy AS, et al.
Clinical predictors of sleep apnea in patients undergoing surgery. Obes Surg 2001;11:28–31.

[15] Jain SS, Dhand R. Perioperative treatment of patients with obstructive sleep apnea. Curr Opin
Pulm Med 2004;10:482–8.

[16] Keeling WB, Haines K, Stone PA, et al. Current indications for preoperative inferior vena cava filter insertion in patients undergoing surgery for morbid
obesity. Obes Surg 2005;15:1009–12.

[17] Gonzales R, Murr M. Predictive factors of venous
thromb-embolic events in patients in patients undergoing Roux-en-Y gastric bypass. Surgery of Obesity
and Related Diseases, in press.

[18] Balsiger BM, Murr MM, Poggio JL, et al. Bariatric
surgery: surgery for weight control in patients with
morbid obesity. Med Clin North Am 2000;84:
477–89.

[19] Nelson L, Gonzalez R, Haines K, et al. Amelioration of gastroesophageal reflux symptoms following
Roux-en-y gastric bypass for clinically significant
obesity. Am Surg 2005;71(11):950–3.

[20] Byrne TK. Complications of surgery for obesity.
Surg Clin North Am 2001;81:1181–93.

[21] Brolin RE, Gorman JH, Gorman RC, et al. Are vitamin B_{12} and folate deficiencies clinically important
after Roux-en-Y gastric bypass. J GI Surg 1998;2:
436–42.

ELSEVIER
SAUNDERS

Perioperative Nursing Clinics 1 (2006) 9–14

PERIOPERATIVE
NURSING
CLINICS

Comorbid Conditions, Patient Criteria, and Costs Associated with Bariatric Surgery

Robin Chard, MSN, RN, CNOR

Florida International University School of Nursing, HLS II-461, 11200 SW 8th Street, Miami, FL 33199, USA

Obesity as defined by the World Health Organization and the National Institutes of Health is measured by the relationship of height to weight, commonly known as "body mass index" (BMI). A person is considered overweight with a BMI of 25 to 29.9 kg/m^2 and obese with BMI of 30 to 39.9 kg/m^2. Morbid obesity is defined as a BMI equal to or greater than 40 kg/m^2 or body weight 100 lb above ideal [1]. With the rising trend of obesity, the numbers of bariatric surgeries has risen significantly as an alternative to managing this prevalent condition. In a recent study funded by the Agency for Health Care Research and Quality, the number of bariatric surgeries in the United States has quadrupled between 1998 and 2002, with a significant increase in costs incurred in treating weight-loss reduction patients [2].

General consensus among practitioners including the National Institutes of Health recommends bariatric surgery for patients with a BMI > 40 kg/m^2 or with BMI > 35 kg/m^2 and one or more significant comorbid conditions, such as cardiovascular disease, sleep apnea, uncontrolled type 2 diabetes, or problems arising during the performance of activities of daily living. Although no studies to date have evaluated the actual recommendations, specialty organizations have developed specific clinical guidelines (Table 1). It is important to note that criteria also include a motivated, compliant patient who has full understanding of the implications both immediate and long-term postprocedure [3].

Because of the plethora of scientific research on obesity treatments, this review of the literature focuses on the comorbid factors, patient selection, and health care costs associated with obesity and bariatric surgery.

Comorbid factors

It is estimated that approximately 300,000 people die of obesity-related deaths annually in the United States; awareness of comorbid conditions is essential when determining candidates for bariatric surgery [4]. Type 2 diabetes, hyperlipidemia, hypertension, obstructive sleep apnea, heart disease, stroke, osteoarthritis, and some cancers, such as endometrial, breast, and colon, are considered some but not all of the comorbid conditions associated with obesity [5]. Collectively, diabetes, hypertension, dyslipidemia, and sleep apnea are considered four of the more important conditions of interest following obesity surgery [6].

In a study of 15,001 adults 25 years and older classified as overweight and obese (BMI ≥25 kg/m^2), the participants possessed several comorbid conditions associated with obesity [7]. The sample for the study was from a previous national survey conducted by the National Center for Health Statistics of the Centers for Disease Control and Prevention. Known as the Third National Health and Nutrition Examination Survey, the focus of the original study was on estimation of the predominance of major diseases, nutritional disorders, and potential risk factors related to obesity found in a representative sample of the United States population. The focus of the follow-up study was to measure the prevalence of conditions identified with obesity by severity, race and ethnicity, and age, including the prevalence of multiple obesity-related comorbidities in the same population. The researchers included high blood

E-mail address: chardr@fiu.edu

Table 1
Clinical guidelines

Organization	Body mass index	Other criteria
National Heart Lung and Blood Institute	BMI >40 or BMI >35 with comorbid conditions	Failure of conventional weight loss therapy
American Gastroenterological Association	BMI >40 or BMI >35 and one or more comorbid conditions (eg, hypertension, heart failure, or sleep apnea)	Failure of conventional weight loss therapy
American College of Preventive Medicine	BMI >40.6	Limit therapy to obese or severely obese

pressure, type 2 diabetes, high blood cholesterol level, coronary heart disease, and gallbladder disease because obesity was previously established as a risk factor for these comorbid conditions.

In general, results indicated that high blood pressure was the most common comorbid condition for men and women, and type 2 diabetes and gallbladder disease increased as weight increased. High blood cholesterol level was very prevalent in both sexes but did not increase in prevalence with increasing weight category. The authors suggested that as obesity continues to rise in the United States, practitioners may become overburdened in treating obesity and the accompanying comorbid conditions. In a study that measured resolution of hypertension and diabetes mellitus following bariatric surgery, 1025 patients were evaluated 1 year postoperative. Hypertension was resolved in 69% and diabetes in 83% of the patients [8].

Obstructive sleep apnea is predominant in many bariatric surgery patients. Researchers evaluated 100 patients postoperatively and found that gastric bypass significantly improved obstructive sleep apnea in most patients [9]. Cholesterol level is an additional comorbid condition in obesity. One study measured the effects of weight regain and lipid levels postsurgery. The researchers found that there was no significant difference among patients who had regained more than or equal to 15% of their lost weight or lost less than 50% of excess weight and patients who maintained a stable weight loss. Findings indicated that normal lipid levels may be long-lasting after bariatric surgery [10].

Obesity is a significant factor in type 2 diabetes and studies indicate that surgery has been the most effective intervention for weight loss and resolution of type 2 diabetes [11]. Buchwald and coworkers [12] conducted a systematic review and meta-analysis of bariatric surgery studies. Data results indicated significant improvements in the comorbid conditions of chronic sleep apnea, hyperlipidemia, type 2 diabetes, and hypertension after bariatric surgery. A different meta-analysis found similar results. Data revealed from 134 studies indicated that diabetes, hypertension, obstructive sleep apnea, and hyperlipidemia had improved or were completely resolved in most patients [13]. Lastly, a review of the evidence on the relationship of obesity surgery and comorbid conditions found either a reduction or resolution of the previously mentioned conditions and additional conditions, such as venous stasis disease, polycystic ovary syndrome, complications of pregnancy and delivery, gastroesophageal reflux disease, stress urinary incontinence, degenerative joint disease, and nonalcoholic steatohepatitis [14].

A prospective Canadian study followed bariatric surgery patients between 1986 and 2002. A cohort of 1035 severely obese patients was matched according to age, length of follow-up, and gender with a control group of 5746 patients who had not undergone surgery. Both groups did not have any significant health-related conditions other than obesity. Follow-up results indicated that the surgical treatment group had significantly reduced their risk for developing cancer, endocrine, cardiovascular, infectious, psychiatric, and mental disorders compared with the control group. No difference was found between the groups relating to hematology conditions and the surgery group had higher risk for digestive disease development [15].

A different prospective study evaluated patients over an 8-year period. Findings indicated that patients who maintained an average weight loss of 40 lb were less likely to develop diabetes mellitus but the weight loss had no long-term effect on hypertension [16].

The Swedish Obesity Study was a large observational nonrandomized study undertaken primarily to report on mortality rates associated with obesity [17]. The Swedish Obesity Study is the only identified study that compared comorbid conditions between surgically treated patients and a concurrent nonsurgical control group. Patients were matched to either surgical or medical treatment groups. It should be noted that patients received a variety of bariatric procedures, such as fixed or variable banding, vertical banded gastroplasty, or gastric bypass. In addition to mortality data, secondary outcome variables were reported on group differences at 2 and 10 years relating to comorbid conditions present in patients at inception, but having no effect on the patients before the surgical or medical treatment for obesity began. A third outcome viewed rate of recovery from risk conditions at 2 and 10 years in patients who were affected at the beginning of the study. The risk conditions considered were blood pressure, serum cholesterol and triglyceride levels, and type 2 diabetes.

At 2- and 10-year rates of recovery, all of the risk factors were lower in the surgical treatment group than in the medical treatment group except for hypercholesterolemia. Patients in the surgical group who had hypertension, diabetes, hypertriglyceridemia, a low high-density lipoprotein cholesterol, and hyperuricemia at baseline had better recoveries than the control group at 2 and 10 years. Hypercholesterolemia rates did not differ among the groups at either 2 or 10 years. In terms of the third outcome variable, the incidence of developing hypertriglyceridemia, diabetes, and hyperuricemia were much lower in the surgical group than in the control group after 2 and 10 years. Low high-density lipoprotein cholesterol was lower in the surgical group at 2 years but not at 10 years. Rates of hypertension and hypercholesterolemia were not different between the groups over the 2- and 10-year periods. Although the study lacked randomization of participants, the data suggested that bariatric surgery was a promising option for obesity and some obesity-relations conditions. In addition to these risk factors, gender was found to be a predictor variable related to life-threatening complications following bariatric surgery [18].

Patient characteristics

Aside from the BMI and comorbid criteria for bariatric surgery, other important considerations should be taken into account as part of patient screening. Patients should fully comprehend the risks and benefits and show a willingness to participate in the postoperative program [19]. Psychosocial factors are heavily weighted because bariatric surgery results in life-long changes for the patient. The American Society for Bariatric Surgery recommends excluding patients who manifest psychopathology that may jeopardize long-term compliance. Other contraindications include active substance abuse and plans to become pregnant within 1 year [20].

One study collected information on whether or not patients were being psychologically evaluated before surgery and what type of evaluation practices were in use. Results indicated that 88% of bariatric programs included psychologic evaluations with approximately 50% using standardized instruments. Common exclusion criteria were active schizophrenia symptoms, mental retardation, illicit drug use, and knowledge deficit related to the procedure. Although the exclusion criteria varied across programs indicating a need for more formalized criteria, most programs did include psychologic testing [21]. Patients need to understand that surgery is not the final chapter in managing obesity but is a part of the on-going maintenance in the weight loss process. Patients may benefit from talking with other individuals who have had the surgery as the lifestyle modifications become a reality postprocedure [22].

Although many variables have been identified in the literature related to patient success after bariatric surgery, few have been established as significant predictors. Relevant variables, such as motivation, socioeconomic status, realistic expectations following surgery, and healthy coping skills, may be related to positive outcomes but in one study were shown to have poor predictor quality [23]. Researchers did conclude in an earlier study that inherent motivational factors did predict ($P < .05$) more weight loss based on scores from the Life Experiences Survey. The authors suggested that preoperative evaluation and intervention may need to be tailored to patients with poorer predictive factors and can be a valuable screening tool [24]. A well-educated patient is essential in ensuring long-term success. Attending classes and support group sessions, making a commitment to follow physician guidelines, and understanding that surgery is not a cure for obesity but one alternative in combating a chronic disease are a few basic needed steps in the process [25]. Implementation of a preoperative behavior modification program was found to be useful in preparing patients for the numerous lifestyle changes needed postsurgery [26].

To evaluate current web sites offering information on bariatric surgery a group of nurse researchers assessed 40 bariatric web sites for exactness and quality. It was concluded that nurses are in a strong position to familiarize themselves with the various web sites and recommend those that have high ratings in quality and accuracy of information [27]. Education for patients and health care providers is key in orchestrating a comprehensive program for potential bariatric patients. At times, individuals are at risk for social stigma regarding their psychologic health associated with being obese and may be considered weak and unable to manage their lives. Health care providers have a unique opportunity to educate themselves regarding obesity in the context of a chronic illness and use their knowledge to facilitate positive patient outcomes [28]. Health care providers face several challenges in caring for obese patients because of their own subtle internal biases directed against obesity. As providers become more aware of the impact of these biases on the caregiver-patient interaction, they may develop more empathetic and healthy relationships with patients [29].

Current thought on the use of bariatric surgery for adolescents is that surgical intervention be recommended only for adolescents who have comorbid conditions and a BMI $\geq 40 \text{ kg/m}^2$. Experts suggest that surgery be considered as an alternative when other conventional treatments have failed. In addition, the potential patient should have a comprehensive preoperative medical and psychologic evaluation [30]. Adolescent bariatric programs should be established within a multidisciplinary format to ensure that optimal management of the course of care carries through the perioperative and long-term follow-up periods [31].

On the opposite end of the spectrum, it has been suggested that patients older than 60 years of age be offered bariatric surgery as an alternative for weight loss. Older patients were shown to have considerable health benefits from surgery comparable with patients less than 60 years of age. Length of stay and postoperative complications were similar for both groups, which offers an additional indicator in support of surgery for older patients [32].

According to the 2000 National Health Interview Survey database, 2.8% of the American population was eligible for obesity surgery in the United States. A disproportionate number of these Americans were undereducated, poor, and black and relied on government health insurance programs, such as Medicare and Medicaid. This may have accounted for a fewer number of blacks undergoing bariatric surgery and that only 13% of bariatric patients in 2000 used Medicare or Medicaid for payment [33]. Race and type of insurance program were variables among 5876 gastric bypass patients in the 2000 National Inpatient Sample Database. Although the variables did not predict postoperative outcomes, it was found that overall costs, length of stay, and incidence of comorbidities were higher in African American patients. Patients enrolled in Medicaid or Medicare insurance programs had longer length of stays, higher mortality and morbidity, and comorbid conditions compared with patients who had private insurance or self-pay formats. Patients with lower incomes had longer length of stays and higher costs [34].

Health care costs and bariatric surgery

The effect of bariatric surgery on health care costs has been the focus of several research studies. A cross-sectional study evaluated pharmaceutical costs between surgical intervention and conventional intervention comparison groups whose participants were from the Swedish Obesity Study. Patients' pharmaceutical needs were followed over a 6-year period. On the average, obese individuals incurred higher medication costs than nonobese individuals but only minimal differences were found between the surgical and conventional weight-loss intervention groups. Although surgical patients had lower expenses for diabetes and cardiovascular disease medications, they had higher costs for gastrointestinal, anemia, and vitamin-deficiency remedies [35].

In another study, researchers analyzed pharmaceutical costs of bariatric surgery patients with the comorbid conditions of hypertension and diabetes preoperatively and at 3- and 9-months postoperatively. A 77.3% reduction occurred in medication costs associated with hypertension and diabetes [36].

An analysis of the costs for bariatric surgery and follow-up treatment among veterans was performed to assess the economic strain on the Veterans Administration health care system. Medical records of 25 postsurgical patients were reviewed and costs calculated over a 12-month period. Results showed that costs of the surgical procedures offset such health care expenses as medications, outpatient visits, and home health devices. It was concluded that resources should be allocated throughout the VA system in support of its existing bariatric surgery programs [37].

Researchers in Quebec found that surgical interventions decrease direct health care costs over a long period of time. A group of surgical patients and a control group were observed over a 5-year period to measure direct health care costs. Although bariatric patients had higher hospital costs, these were offset by the reduction over time of additional health care costs [38].

One study specifically looked at the relationship between laparoscopic gastric bypass and monthly prescription costs at preoperative and postoperative intervals. Because of the improved comorbid conditions of gastroesophageal reflux disease, hypertension, diabetes, and hypercholesterolemia, patients had an overall mean monthly decrease in prescription costs within 6 months. Costs did not include over-the-counter nutritional supplements, such as vitamins [39]. From the payer perspective, researchers found that bariatric surgery was more cost-effective than no treatment for severely obese patients [40]. The presence of comorbid conditions, such as type 2 diabetes and sleep apnea, and postoperative complications were found to increase hospital costs for bariatric surgery patients [41].

Summary

It is an unfortunate fact that obesity has become an epidemic in the United States. Greater than 60% of the population is now either overweight or obese [42]. Numerous reasons are attributed to why diet, medications, and lifestyle changes have failed to curb this alarming trend. To treat obesity and the comorbid conditions associated with the disease, bariatric surgery has been shown to be effective in reducing immediate and long-term weight loss. Past and future researchers will continue to pursue evidence relating to predictor variables associated with bariatric surgery, the most safe and effective techniques, and cost analyses.

References

[1] Sammons D. Roux-en-Y gastric bypass: a surgical treatment for morbid obesity. Am J Nurs 2002; 102:24A.

[2] Encinosa W, Bernard M, Steiner C, et al. Use and costs of bariatric surgery and prescription weight-loss medications. Health Aff (Millwood) 2005;24: 1039–46.

[3] Dowden C. What are the indications for bariatric surgery? J Fam Pract 2005;54:633–43.

[4] Allison D, Fontaine K, Manson JA, et al. Annual deaths attributable to obesity in the United States. JAMA 1999;282:1530–8.

[5] Must A, Spadano J, Coakley E, et al. The disease burden associated with overweight and obesity. JAMA 1999;282:1523–9.

[6] Maggard M, Shugarman L, Suttorp M, et al. Meta-analysis: surgical treatment of obesity. Ann Intern Med 2005;142:547–59.

[7] Centers for Disease Control and Prevention. Overweight and obesity: home. Available at: http://www.cdc.gov/nccdphp/dnpa/obesity. Accessed September 12, 2005.

[8] Sugerman HJ, Wolfe LG, Sica DA, et al. Diabetes and hypertension in severe obesity and effects of gastric bypass-induced weight loss. Ann Surg 2003;237: 751–8.

[9] Rasheid S, Banasiak M, Gallagher SF, et al. Gastric bypass is an effective treatment for obstructive sleep apnea in patients with clinically significant obesity. Obes Surg 2003;13:58–61.

[10] Brolin RE, Bradley LJ, Wilson AC, et al. Lipid risk profile and weight stability after gastric restrictive operations for morbid obesity. J Gastrointest Surg 2000;4:464–9.

[11] Cornier M. Obesity and diabetes. Curr Opin Endocrinol Diabetes 2005;12:260–6.

[12] Buchwald H, Avidor Y, Braunwald E, et al. Bariatric surgery: a systematic review and meta-analysis. JAMA 2004;292:1724–37.

[13] Overweight, obesity, and health risk: National Task Force on the Prevention and Treatment of Obesity. Arch Intern Med 2000;160:898–904.

[14] Lara MD, Kothari S, Sugerman HJ. Surgical management of obesity: a review of the evidence relating to the health benefits and risks. Treat Endocrinol 2005;4:55–64.

[15] Christou NV, Sampalis JS, Liberman M, et al. Surgery decreases long-term mortality, morbidity, and health care use in morbidly obese patients. Ann Surg 2004;240:416–24.

[16] Sjöström CD, Peltonen M, Wedel H, et al. Differentiated long-term effects of intentional weight loss on diabetes and hypertension. Hypertension 2000; 36:20.

[17] Sjostrom L, Lindroos AK, Peltonen M, et al. Lifestyle, diabetes, and cardiovascular risk factors 10 years after bariatric surgery. N Engl J Med 2004; 351:2683–93.

[18] Livingston EH, Huerta S, Arthur D, et al. Male gender is a predictor of morbidity and age a predictor of mortality for patients undergoing gastric bypass surgery. Ann Surg 2002;236:576–82.

[19] Gallagher S. Taking the weight off with bariatric surgery. Nursing (Brux) 2004;34:58–64.

[20] American Society for Bariatric Surgery. Rationale for the surgical treatment of morbid obesity.

Available at: http://www.asbs.org/html/patients/
rationale.html. Accessed September 12, 2005.

[21] Bauchowitz A, Gonder-Frederick L, Olbrisch M,
et al. Psychosocial evaluation of bariatric surgery
candidates: a survey of present practices. Psychosom
Med 2005;67:825–32.

[22] Alexander N. Surgical management of obesity. Clin
Obstet Gynecol 2004;47:928–41.

[23] van Hout GC, Verschure SK, van Heck GL. Psychosocial predictors of success following bariatric surgery. Obes Surg 2005;15:552–60.

[24] Ray E, Nickels M, Sayeed S, et al. Predicting success
after gastric bypass: the role of psychosocial and behavioral factors. Surgery 2003;134:555–64.

[25] Ryan MA. My story: a personal perspective on bariatric surgery. Crit Care Nurs Q 2005;28:288–92.

[26] Brandenburg D, Kotlowski R. Practice makes per-
fect? Patient response to a prebariatric surgery behavior modification program. Obes Surg 2005;15:
125–32.

[27] Nichols C, Oermann MH. An evaluation of bariatric
web sites for patient education and guidance. Gastroenterol Nurs 2005;28:112–7.

[28] Murray D. Morbid obesity-psychosocial aspects and
surgical interventions. AORN J 2003;78:990–5.

[29] Reto CS. Psychological aspects of delivering nursing
care to the bariatric patient. Crit Care Nurs Q 2003;
26:139–49.

[30] Durant N, Cox J. Current treatment approaches to
overweight in adolescents. Curr Opin Pediatr 2005;
17:454–9.

[31] Warman JL. The application of laparoscopic bariatric surgery for treatment of severe obesity in adolescents using a multidisciplinary adolescent
bariatric program. Crit Care Nurs Q 2005;28:
276–87.

[32] St Peter S, Craft R, Tiede J, et al. Impact of advanced age on weight loss and health benefits after

laparoscopic gastric bypass. Arch Surg 2005;140:
165–8.

[33] Carbonell AM, Lincourt AE, Matthews BD, et al.
National study of the effect of patient and hospital
characteristics on bariatric surgery outcomes. Am
Surg 2005;71:308–14.

[34] Livingston E, Ko CY. Socioeconomic characteristics of the population eligible for obesity surgery.
Surgery 2004;135:288–96.

[35] Narbro K, Agren G, Jonsson E, et al. Pharmaceutical costs in obese individuals: comparison with a ran-
domly selected population sample and long-term
changes after conventional and surgical treatment:
the SOS intervention study. Arch Intern Med 2002;
162:2061–9.

[36] Potteiger CE, Paragi PR, Inverso NA, et al. Bariatric
surgery: shedding the monetary weight of prescription costs in the managed care arena. Obes Surg
2004;14:725–30.

[37] Gallagher SF, Banasiak M, Gonzalvo JP, et al. The
impact of bariatric surgery on the Veterans Administration healthcare system: a cost analysis. Obes
Surg 2003;13:245–8.

[38] Sampalis JS, Liberman M, Auger S, et al. The impact of weight reduction surgery on health-care costs
in morbidly obese patients. Obes Surg 2004;14:
939–47.

[39] Gould JC, Garren MJ, Starling JR. Laparoscopic
gastric bypass results in decreased prescription medication costs within 6 months. J Gastrointest Surg
2004;8:983–7.

[40] Fang J. The cost-effectiveness of bariatric surgery.
Am J Gastroenterol 2003;98:2097–8.

[41] Cooney RN, Haluck RS, Ku J, et al. Analysis of cost
outliers after gastric bypass surgery: what can we
learn? Obes Surg 2003;13:29–36.

[42] O'Connell TL. An overview of obesity and weight
loss surgery. Clinical Diabetes 2004;22:115–20.

ELSEVIER SAUNDERS

Perioperative Nursing Clinics 1 (2006) 15–23

PERIOPERATIVE NURSING CLINICS

Prejudice, Bias, and Stigma: Inevitable Factors that Impact Bariatric Treatment

Rita C. Scheidt, RNC, BSN

Department of Continuing Education and Staff Development, MedCentral Health System, 335 Glessner Avenue, Mansfield, OH 44903, USA

Prejudice is opinion without judgment.
Voltaire (1694–1778) [1]

Obesity has a human face. Whether on a short jaunt around any shopping mall, an excursion to a sporting event, an evening at the theater, a visit to a homeless shelter or health clinic, or a walk through the corridors of a hospital, it is evident that a large part of the population are far from what is considered normal weight according to current body mass index (BMI) tables. The culture in which we live places a high value on physical beauty. Thinness is high on the list of desirable attributes. An article published in 2001 reports the results of a survey asking whether physical beauty or inner beauty counts more in the real world. "One third of the participants over the age of 18 said that they thought, 'physical beauty' counts more." One fourth of women respondents considered keeping an attractive appearance "essential," and "more than half said that they considered it at least 'important'" [2]. The culture admires well-chiseled men and prizes women who are thin and have a youthful body. Thin is in; obesity is out.

Ideas of what is beautiful have changed over the ages much like fashion. It has been said that art imitates life. A brief look at the art of the past shows that Rubens and Renoir painted women subjects who were obese, or at least overweight by today's standards. Did this indicate a preference for a more ample body size? Stunkard and co-workers [3] suggest that perhaps these paintings are more indicative the patron's preference rather than the reality of the societal norm of the day.

Although far removed from the time of Rubens and Renoir, the article seems to connect the roots of bias against obesity then and now in Western culture to the Biblical admonition against gluttony. Although the Biblical canon may lead one to such a conclusion, it is also just as likely that gluttony refers to all manner of overindulgence or excess that extends beyond food intake.

Women today, especially young girls, struggle with body image issues, as evidenced by the increasingly large numbers of eating disorders, such as anorexia and bulimia, reported in both popular and medical literature. The phenomenon affects both genders and extends across all races and ethnicities. Most recently, older women are succumbing to disordered eating behaviors to ensure a svelte figure. Many believe that how images, particularly female, are portrayed in the media has a considerable impact on how women view their bodies [4].

A discussion with a young woman who has struggled with body image issues, how obesity and her spirituality connect, demonstrates the considerable challenge this subject can be for some. Rebecca is 22 years old and a college student. She describes herself as a "yoyo dieter." She is a Christian who seeks an authentic faith. She has not hesitated to question traditional beliefs. She noted that when she was obese, a BMI of 35, she felt excluded from others in her small group that met once a week for Bible study and prayer. The group advocated the idea that being overweight was a direct result of, or a simple matter of, disobedience to God's will. Obesity, evidence of gluttony, which is one of the seven deadly sins, is proof positive of a sinful life. Rebecca felt guilty and in need of repentance and cleansing.

E-mail address: jscheidt@neo.rr.com

doi:10.1016/j.cpen.2005.12.002

Although no one directly confronted her, the feeling that she was "living in sin" continued. She felt increasingly excluded, and it hurt. This motivated her to embark on a strict weight loss program. She lost weight and as the pounds melted away, she took pleasure in the way she looked. She was pleased with her progress and assumed that her interactions with the group would improve; they did. She was welcomed and affirmed in her victory over iniquity. This state of acceptance was short lived when a new pastor arrived. His perspective was quite different. The pastoral stance that people who go to great lengths to stay thin focus on the externals seemed to catapult Rebecca's into the opposite direction. She said the experience deeply affected her. Rebecca had the distinct impression that she was focusing too much on her body, she had turned too far in the direction toward self-improvement. Now Rebecca thought herself guilty of vainglory and not spiritual enough. As a result, Rebecca continued to feel like an outsider, that she did not fit. This experience is not unique and one can easily see how such encounters can be confusing and injurious.

Art, films, and especially television of today promote the culture of thinness with great finesse. A study in 2003 investigated the "distribution and individual characteristics on prime-time television" [5]. Some have called it "fat bias" and according to research is the experience of many, if not most obese individuals. Some have identified the prejudice against obese or overweight people as the "last socially acceptable form of prejudice." In current culture, sexism, racism, anti-Semitism, and lately the mistrust of people of Arab descent is culturally inappropriate. The public forum is quick to point out the unjust marginalization of women, African Americans, Jews, and Arabs. When it comes to obesity, however, social norms represent a different standard of tolerance. Prejudice against the overweight and obese is socially acceptable, supported, and promoted in a variety of media [6].

Television, movies, comedians, magazines, and newspapers often contain material that is clearly offensive to the obese. For example, *Shallow Hal*, a movie starring Gweneth Paltrow who donned a "fat suit" for the movie, featured content that mocked obesity, using it as a basis for comedy. The point of the whole movie was to make a statement about superficiality. Yet, throughout, by using sight gags and tricks of the camera, the movie succeeded in using obesity as the object of derision. Perhaps the intention of the film was to show unfair treatment of overweight individuals; it was unambiguous. The jokes and visual gags that showed the svelte Paltrow vacillating from her thin frame into a bulging fat woman were attempts at high comedy that achieved little more than a grotesque and visually distasteful demonstration of fat bias [6]. It is true that researchers repeatedly imply or state that television and other media (film, photography, and print) have the capacity to promote the negative characterization of the obese, if only by emphasizing the thin as desirable and ideal.

Television regularly portrays a host of negative depictions of overweight individuals, both men and women of all ages, races, and ethnicities who are plus-sized. Comedians in their comedy routines regularly poke fun at the size, shape, eating habits, and dating prospects of the obese. Negative characteristics are regularly attributed to the obese more often than to thin people. Greenberg and coworkers [5] used a number of variables in conducting their research to authenticate their theses, and their research found that there is a verifiable neglect of overweight individuals and a demonstrated favoritism in who gets which parts, whether the thin or obese get the major roles. Television promotes negative stereotypical attributions toward overweight and obesity and reflects to an accurate degree the experience of the obese in society. The research shows views commonly expressed in that the obese are "undisciplined, dishonest, sloppy, ugly, socially unattractive, sexually unskilled, and less likely to do productive work." The danger of the perpetuation of such stereotypes in relation to any identified group, be they African American, Hispanic, female, or other ethnic group, is that when the media present them with such disdain and derision, the implication is that these groups are less valued, marginalized, and trivial. The media contributes to the stigma associated with not only the obese, but also with other segments of the population that are judged inferior or less desirable.

Balko [7], a policy analyst with the Cato Institute, quotes Surgeon General Richard Caromona: "As we look to the future and where childhood obesity will be in 20 years...it is every bit as threatening as is the terrorist threat we face today. It is the threat from within." He goes on to include a poll that stated that "almost 90% of Americans put the blame for obesity on individuals who are obese." He goes on to state that "obesity ought to be a matter of private concern and not public policy, that overweight may not be the dire condition some say it is, or that data suggesting we're all ballooning to plus sizes may be misleading, are points the media won't even take into consideration." The association or connection between terrorism and obesity may be somewhat reckless or imprudent.

On a Medscape General Medicine web cast video editorial, Lundberg [8] offered a solution to the obesity epidemic. In his first of three, called "How to prevent the obese from becoming 'obeser'–stop eating," he delivered a diatribe of accusations, innuendo, and negative commentary. He stated, "How can we stop the obese from becoming more obese? Pretty simple. Stop feeding them." He connects various "self-destructive" behaviors and infers similarity or likeness: we seek to prevent drunk drivers from driving, we ticket speeders, level penalties, and put a great deal of effort in preventing exposure to addicting drugs and tobacco. Nevertheless, he says, "An obese person enters an eating joint, or a supermarket, and buys and eats any and everything he or she wants, and nobody seems to care." He does not fail to point the finger at all those elements of society that profit from the plight of the obese. He levels accusations of profiteering at pharmaceutical companies, science, genetics, surgery, nutrition, fast food, companies that make soft drinks, vending machine companies, those who hawk exercise programs and aerobics classes, and even school boards.

This same physician continued his conjecture, acknowledging that he stirred up a "firestorm" in that there were 200 letters to the editor. Of the 200, 78 were supportive, 65 disagreed, and 56 were classified as neutral. He apologized for his "satire" [9]. On careful reading of these responses, it is doubtful that he grasped the impact of his faux pas. His claim of satire was clearly a defensive response. On viewing this segment several times, it was not clear that he meant to be funny. His demeanor was serious and the expression on his face, the inflection and tone of his voice marked him as a physician "in the know" proclaiming the "truth." In this second web cast, he repeated his "stop eating" mockery several times. He extended his version of the "blame game" to the "enablers of obesity" [9]. The doctor did not identify the enablers.

Lundberg's [10] third web cast is an attempt to analyze. He highlights some of the responses he received. Again, his effort at humor falls flat. He stated that because of the many responses to his web casts, and because of the strong interest in clinical nutrition and obesity, Medscape had initiated an eSection just for those special interests.

It is evident that the medical community as a whole has a challenge. Health care providers need to sift through the research and strive for a balanced and therapeutic response to the problem of obesity if professionals intend to provide health care that is both compassionate and focused on health promotion, rather than promoting body types and defining beauty. This is important because the medical community is not immune from the prejudice and bias that is upsetting to many Americans.

In 2003, a study funded by the Rudd Institute, a nonprofit foundation whose purpose is to study antifat bias, examined the antifat bias among health professionals specializing in obesity treatment. The study's lead author Marlene B. Schwartz, coordinator of the Yale Center for Eating and Weight Disorders, was interviewed by Medscape Medical News. She stated that the study found a significant level of automatic antifat bias among health professionals who specialize in obesity; it was lower than results of earlier research, but the presence of this bias continues. Her opinion indicates that although health professionals were less biased than lay people, they were biased. Research shows the power of the stigma and the strong grip the tendency to stereotype is in the culture. She maintained that the purpose of the study was broader than to identify the antibias of health care professionals serving the obese population, but to explore ways to combat the bias and promote "positive attitudes toward obese individuals" [11].

The findings of this study are disturbing. Participants in the study agreed with the generally accepted opinion that the obese are lazy, stupid, and worthless. In addition, this perception holds despite realizing that obesity is caused by a multitude of factors, among which are genetic and environmental. Obesity is not primarily a result of the behavior of the individual, or evidence of a grave character flaw. The bias is so deep that it includes negative assumptions about the intelligence and personal worth of the obese. In caring for patients, if the bias is present, the study suggests that it may result in substandard treatment that may include less time spent with patients, minimal empathy, poor interaction, and less emphasis on an optimistic outlook for progress. It may result in a reduced willingness to provide the support patients need [12].

The study cites other research that surveyed obese patients, and nearly two thirds indicated that their experiences with physicians suggest that they believe that their care providers generally do not comprehend the hardships they encounter [12]. The evidence of this bias toward the obese extends to other members of health care professions. The study refers to a survey of nurses in which 28% indicated that they felt repulsion at the sight of a person who is obese. A similar survey of 438 doctors named obesity as the fifth most negative patient feature. The American Academy of Family Physicians surveyed 324 members, and of these 39% believed that obese patients were lazy and two thirds thought that obese patients lacked self-control. Some surveys exploring physicians' attitudes demonstrated that when doctors described obese patients they used words like "weak-willed," "ugly," and "awkward." Most patients who seek weight-loss surgery report disrespectful treatment from primary health care providers [12].

A study of the attitudes of exercise science students, done through the Centers for Integrated Health Research, concludes that "...students in the field of exercise science possess negative associations and bias toward obese individuals" [13]. The correlation with the bias found in the other groups is a strong one, and this may contribute to negative experiences of the obese and may have a negative impact on efforts at health promotion by further alienating those who most need the services.

A study done at Duke University Medical Center found that obese or overweight people may not get the preventative health care they need. There was a positive correlation between increasing BMI and a reduced number of mammograms and Pap smears. A startling fact cited is that, "a white woman of normal weight was more than 50% more likely to receive a mammogram than a severely obese woman." The researchers put forward the supposition that perhaps the reason for this lack of preventative health care may be the pervasive prevalence of stigma and bias attributed to the obese patient by health care providers [14].

Another article on the Weight-control Information, a site promoted by the National Institutes of Health, discusses research done by the University of Pennsylvania's School of Medicine about the attitudes of primary care physicians that concurred with the findings of other researchers [15]. They indicate that often the anticipation that

they will be treated with disrespect leads obese patients to avoid going to their physicians. Six hundred and twenty physicians were sent questionnaires about their opinions about obesity treatment. More than 50% reported that they "...viewed patients who are obese as awkward, unattractive, ugly and not compliant. One-third described such patients as weak-willed, sloppy or lazy." A significant number believe that "treatment for obesity is ineffective." The article concludes that a more considerate style when helping obese patients in their struggle with weight is a good starting point in approaching the "obesity epidemic." The serious consequences of obesity and the health issues involved make this discrimination especially destructive, because obese people often have an increased need for medical attention. Avoiding or delaying medical attention in light of the comorbidities of obesity is unsafe. Not getting the care they need, for some, may mean an early death.

In interviewing nurses who are obese and persistently struggle with obesity, they agree that stigma and prejudice make a significant contribution to their own sense of well-being and self-worth. When nurses care for the obese patient, it is not uncommon to hear derogatory remarks about the patient. Although not made within hearing of the obese patient, one can assume that such strong culturally supported bias is difficult to mask and may have a negative impact on patient care.

In an adolescent inpatient psychiatric unit, when a patient was obese, in nearly every instance they were the object of ridicule and disparaging, hateful remarks. The treatment challenge to nursing staff effectively to ameliorate the damage done was to find ways of communicating with the injured adolescent in a therapeutic way. Often, little could be done to move the patient toward improvement of self-image and toward a realistic and reasonable body image that could have a positive effect on their treatment.

Patients who have battled obesity most of their lives, go on diet after diet, join Weight Watchers, attend Overeaters Anonymous meetings, and endure the prejudice and stereotyping common to the culture sometimes choose bariatric surgery. Most of the time this choice is a last resort; they are simply tired of trying to "become normal." Many have been the object of ridicule in their own families, often becoming the scapegoat for family conflict. Stories abound; books, both fiction and nonfiction, have been written that confirm the experience of the obese as marginalized and maligned.

The experience of a 24-year-old woman who is obese is common. Paula had been a "chubby" baby. She poured over family picture albums and saw for herself, even as a baby she was fat, there was no denying it. She had sought help from her family physician who admonished her to quit "killing herself" and gave her a prescription for a tricyclic antidepressant and mood elevator. Her mother told her repeatedly, "how could you do this to me," indicating that she was ashamed of what the neighbors and the people at church would think. In fact, at the age of 11 her mother had taken her to the family doctor who sympathized with the mother's exasperation and frustration about her endless efforts to make her daughter lose weight. He prescribed thyroid extract and amphetamines. For several years, Paula took amphetamines as prescribed and lost weight. She did not experience the nervousness and other negative side effects. Anticipating her high school graduation, she was ecstatic and thought herself to be "normal." She was overjoyed that she would be able to wear a beautiful, size 13 junior, white dress to her high school graduation. After graduation and going off amphetamines, she slowly regained the weight and then some. Her father poked fun at her. He reminded her that as a baby the chubbiness was cute, a sign of health. He taunted her by singing, "Honey you were a beautiful baby, but look at you now." Paula lived alone, had a job, and went to work to pay the bills. When not at work, she isolated herself. She gained more and more weight. She felt guilty, angry, and hopeless— a failure. Now, at age 24, she weighed 230 pounds and contemplated suicide. Then she learned about bariatric surgery.

Paula made an appointment with the surgeon and began her journey through the maze that unfolds before every patient who seeks this surgery. Whether one agrees or disagrees about the appropriateness of the patient's choice, to go on severe calorie-restricted diets, enlist in a weight-loss program, or choose to have bariatric surgery, the choice remains the patient's. Health care providers must honor the patient's decision. To do so promotes patient autonomy and the patient's right to self-determination. Paula had to submit to the many requirements, preoperative testing, examinations, and counseling to ensure that she was an appropriate candidate for the gastric bypass. These hoops are necessary. They help the physician to provide every opportunity for a positive and satisfying outcome that is long-term success because of the surgical intervention. Insurance companies require this in-depth assessment of the patient to determine whether they reimburse for part or all of the procedure.

People are choosing to have bariatric surgery more frequently. According to a study from the Agency for Health Care Research and Quality, between 1998 and 2002, bariatric surgeries increased in number from 13,386 to 71,733. That is five times as many as in 2002. A major part of this increase was the large number of patients between 55 and 64 who had the operation [16].

The new American College of Physicians guidelines target obesity management. Quotes from the online version of the ACP Observer cite that in 2003 there were 103,200 bariatric surgeries, and in 2004 there were 140,640. The American College of Physicians now recommends surgery for those who are severely obese. These figures indicate a significant rise in the frequency of bariatric surgery. This does not imply that choosing bariatric surgery is easier or less complicated for the individual. In 2004, Medicare for the first time conceded that obesity is a disease. Yet the agency does not cover physician-supervised obesity treatment; nor does it cover bariatric surgery unless it is part of treatment for comorbidities. Few insurance carriers reimburse for obesity management, which may include diet, medication, exercise programs, and counseling [17].

The number of articles, books, and research papers that address obesity is staggering. Popular magazines, newspapers, and electronic media are filled with information, some accurate, some unmistakably tabloid. The Department of Health Human Services, the Office of the Surgeon General, has issued grave warnings about the "obesity epidemic," how Americans must take greater responsibility for their own health [18]. The body of scientific knowledge about obesity is vast. There is research to support nearly every perspective on obesity, its management, and causes; comorbidities; the relationship between BMI and increasing morbidity; and the specter of an early death.

Several recently published books challenge much of the current research and reach very different, if not contradictory conclusions. They offer alternative viewpoints and different conclusions. Often these are critical of the cultural momentum fueled by research that is perhaps flawed or incomplete. In one controversial book that is well worth examining, Gard and Wright [19] suggest that current research and the general media offer a somewhat hazy compilation of information that is laden with moral schema and ideological conjecture. The work is analytical and thought provoking. It challenges traditional medical and scientific wisdom and the firmly held beliefs that accompany them. Campos [20] identifies the questionable aspects of the "war on obesity," the science, and the political and cultural significance of weight. He then presents a balanced and reasoned antidote to the fixation, which he believes is hurting people more than helping. His book has the support of a number of researchers in obesity.

The National Institutes of Health in guidelines for the treatment of obesity in adults define obesity as "a complex, multifactorial disease that develops from the interaction between genotype and the environment. Our understanding of how and why obesity occurs is incomplete; however, it involves the integration of social, behavioral, cultural, physiological, metabolic, and genetic factors" [18]. From this definition one can see that the understanding exemplified by this definition is not conclusive, nor is it blatantly indicative of any one causative agent. There is much to learn about obesity. Health care professionals need to learn and then educate patients and community. This is important, especially if one wants to provide supportive interactions and medical guidance with sensitivity.

The decision to have bariatric surgery involves many aspects, factors, and pressures. The choice for surgery is often the last of many treatment decisions. Each patient's experience is unique and distinct. Each patient has a story to tell. The experience common to all patients who are overweight or obese is the firmly entrenched prejudice that impinges on every aspect of their lives. Their stories, if heard and understood, might serve to stimulate a level of empathy that augments the efforts of health care providers to provide the kind of help and support needed to reduce it. A collection of essays promoting the use of story in the practice of medicine and ethical decision-making includes a quote from a novel by Shem. The paragraph illustrates how when a physician looks beyond the body, the patient become a person, and empathy is born [21].

I realized how much my vision had broadened. Instead of seeing just bodies, I was seeing people, reading people, sensing in people's faces, postures,

and words and in the intangible stuff, some truth about the person, not only in terms of each life, but in each as part of any life, of life itself. I saw the sorrow behind the smile, the years of pain pulling out the lines from the corners of the mouth and eyes, the rage provoking the scar, the weight of nostalgia tugging down the lip, even the smile behind the sorrow. From my year of focusing on the something else besides what these people were showing me consciously, they had become more translucent yet more substantial, in the way that the translucency of a deep-sea creature reveals the bones, the guts, the feathery beat of the heart, that glassy-ribbed heart.

Paula had the bariatric surgery and did well. She has adjusted and made the necessary lifestyle changes that have allowed her to maintain a loss of 75 pounds for 3 years. Today she reports that she would do it all over again. She exercises regularly and the diet she is on is satisfying for her. Her days of diet drugs, shame, and depression are over. She validates the research cited here, in that she experienced the bias and disrespect before surgery, but now that she has lost weight, she no longer feels that she is disrespected or mistreated. She has a positive level of self-esteem and healthy body image.

Other patients are not so lucky. The complications that may follow bariatric surgery can be devastating. Some can be as simple as a mild fever that lingers or an occasional bout of the "dumping syndrome." Other experiences begin with bariatric surgery and end up with multiple surgeries to correct complications, such as postoperative infections and hernias. Oelschlager [22] lists the major complications of bariatric surgery from a gastroenterologist's perspective: (1) stricture of the gastrojejunostomy (5%–10%); (2) gastrointestinal bleeding (1%–2%); (3) marginal ulcers on the gastric side of the gastrojejunostomy; (4) bowel obstruction caused by adhesions; and (5) following LapBand, migration of the band, severe food intolerance, and gastroesophageal reflux. He goes on to say that as the number of bariatric surgeries increase gastroenterologists need to be aware of these complications to provide the care these patients need.

A woman recently shared that a dear friend of hers had bariatric surgery, lost all the weight she anticipated, and says that despite the medical problems she now faces, she feels so "good" about herself. This woman has had several surgeries since the original bariatric procedure, has had several serious infections, and now may need dialysis for the rest of her life. Her friend, sad and empathetic, said that she wished her friend had stayed fat.

Another way to talk about the care and treatment of the bariatric patient is to recognize bariatric patients as a group, as a culture. This makes it an issue of cultural diversity. Cultural competence is a necessary component in health care and any service-oriented business. Health care facilities include diversity training in orientation programs and regular features of in-service training programs. That patients who are obese represent a culture is substantial. There is a proliferation of support groups, an increasing number of weight loss programs, fitness clubs, and one new diet after another. On the Internet, one finds discussion groups that focus on weight management, and the swapping of recipes, the latest imitation of some forbidden food that tastes like the real thing at half the calories. There are many web sites disseminating information for obesity treatment centers, basic health information geared to the overweight, list servers, and blogs. These reflect the same kind of development in print media. There are activist organizations, groups that promote "fat acceptance," and web sites hosted by organizations working to educate about bias and stigma to change minds and influence public opinion. The plethora of information may not be applicable to all patients. Health care professionals are in a good position to guide patients to sites that contain reliable information and are trustworthy.

The idea that obesity is a diversity issue was evident when visiting a chat room for patients who are interested in, are anticipating, or have had bariatric surgery. On entering the chat room, a question posted was, "Have any of you decided against bariatric surgery and why"? No one answered for some time, then finally a participant stated, "We are all pro bariatric surgery." That was the only response, but the chatter continued about how each was doing, how much weight they had lost, how good they felt, and how proud they were. Some asked questions like, "Were you scared? My surgery is next week and I am scared"? The mutual support and encouragement was consistently positive. The observation validated that there also is bias and prejudice within the community of the obese; they too are not immune from the cultural trends that drive the phenomena of bias and prejudice. When one asked about nonsurgical treatment, also a valid choice, the support was noticeably lacking.

This is a litigious society. Note the pervasive litany of lawsuits publicized by the media. An airline company is sued because they tried to force an obese person to buy two tickets. There are discussions of who has the responsibility for obesity caused by a high intake of super-sized meals in a lawsuit against McDonald's for aiding and abetting obesity. On August 23, 2005, several networks presented a news story that marked yet another dimension of this complex issue. A physician went public with the fact that a woman offended by his advice concerning her obesity filed a complaint with the medical board of New Hampshire. The woman stated that his advice was, "hurtful and not helpful." The medical board has launched an investigation and now the attorney general's office is involved. The doctor stated that he had written a letter of apology. He defended himself by saying that he was only doing his job [23]. This is not much different from saying. "I was only following orders."

After viewing the interview several times, it was clear that bias and prejudice was clearly a factor. It is reasonable for a physician to provide information and guidance concerning weight issues, and to promote healthy lifestyle change. This physician stated that he began to give the patient information about obesity and began to list the dangers and peril she would face if she did not change. Mid-list the physician stated, "By this time, they usually break down...but she didn't break down...." Was the physician's goal to "break her down"? If so, this is yet another stark example of the insensitivity described in the research that is reviewed here [23].

Negative attitudes and beliefs about the obese have been a part of culture for a long time. The root of the phenomena extends beyond the scope of this article. Perhaps one of the most damaging beliefs is that those who are overweight or obese are directly responsible for their condition: the idea that "they brought it on themselves," or "well you get what you deserve," or the folksy "you are what you eat." Such beliefs may lead to the perception that ones' weight is under conscious control and point to a fact that the obese have abandoned all good taste and chosen to be obese. The statement "how could anyone let themselves get like that" is often said with a forced tone of pity that contains within it the accusation: the person has no will power or self-control. One would surmise that among mental health care professionals, the obese person would find some level of empathy, and some do. Yet, one woman shared that her therapist told her to take the pictures her doctor gave her after an esophagoscopy diagnostic of reflux disease (they showed the bright red lining of her stomach oozing blood) and tape them to the sun visor of her car, or near the speedometer to help her to avoid stopping in fast food restaurants. In the mental health care field, obese clients time after time are rated as lower functioning than clients of normal weight. Obesity is often identified as the stain of personal failure born of a serious character flaw.

Health care professionals, physicians, nurses, laboratory employees, clinics, or receptionists in doctor's offices should reflect on personal perceptions and beliefs about obesity and overweight. Learn the difference between fact and truth. A person may weigh more than the BMI tables outline: that is a fact. The truth, however, is that there may be reasons for which science and medicine have no concrete explanation. Obesity has a face. Empathy not sympathy or pity serve this population well. Recognize the value judgments made automatically, without considering reality.

Listen to the conversation around you, when someone is on a diet and eats something calorific, they often say, "I've been bad." When they eat a salad with fat-free and sugar-free salad dressing they are proud that "They've been good." Recognize that the culture, no matter how enlightened, is conditioned to idealize thinness and demonize those with more weight than insurance tables allow.

Ask yourself, "How do I see myself"? Moreover, "What conclusions do I make about my clients or patients"? Do your thoughts automatically align with the bias and prejudice illustrated by the research? Do you fall into the trap of blaming the patient? Are bariatric patients harder to care for, more difficult to understand, empathize with, or even like? One should consider these questions and as one encounters overweight and obese patients, exercise a level of self-reflection that leads to a higher level of self-awareness. Only in this way will one make progress in providing compassionate and quality care.

Bariatric patients have bought into some of the same biases and perceptions and internalized the damaging effects. This further inhibits their health-seeking behaviors. They may feel embarrassment and a level of shame unimaginable to the uninformed health care provider. It is natural for them, as they come for bariatric surgery, to have serious doubt about their decision to have the procedure. Although many have researched and explored all the ins and outs of bariatric surgery, they still are subject to the fear that "all will not be well" after surgery. Go to the web site http://www.obesityhelp.com/morbidobesity/wlsmemorial.phtml and view the list of those who did not make it [24]. The choice for surgery is not an easy one to make.

One must remember that, even though the consequences may be negative, these patients feel hope, expectation, and excitement about what they believe will be a better and healthier life. It is common for patients to wonder if this will be another in a long list of failures. No matter how one views the matter, from whatever perspective, the choice for bariatric surgery is not the easy way out. Living large in a culture that worships thinness is not easy living.

Suggestions that may assist in caring for an obese patient, whether they come for bariatric surgery or an external fixation of a fractured wrist include being respectful. Refrain from making remarks that indicate hesitation in communicating with them. When taking care of a person struggling with weight issues, maintain professional boundaries. Imagine how insulting it is for a nurse to share her personal struggle with weight with a person twice her size. Strive for every opportunity to show empathy and not pity. Do not question their decision, respect it; it is professional behavior, compassion interaction, and ethical medical management.

When providing patient care, anticipate their needs. Does your facility stock large patient gowns, blood pressure cuffs, or have other equipment that makes giving patient care safer and more comfortable for the patient? Note the size of the chairs in the waiting area. Often, family members are also large. Noticing the "small" things is part of customer service that meets the needs of both patient and family.

All patients, large or small, are sensitive to the communication between staff members as they go about their work. In speaking with nurses about the care of bariatric patients, they report that often staff members shy away from caring for them, for fear of hurting themselves. The application of correct body mechanics and having enough help prevents injury. A patient once shared that when called on to assist in moving a large patient, the primary caregiver rolled their eyes and sighed. Experiencing the stigma in such a profound way was hurtful. Be aware that even subtle unconscious actions may communicate the negative bias one wants to avoid. Recognize that patients who have experienced and lived with bias and discrimination are sensitive to even minimal signs of it. Patients turn to the medical community for help. It is in the medical community where strides toward a reduction of stigma and discrimination must begin.

References

[1] Famous Quotes: Voltaire. Available at: http://www.mothers4peace.org/famous%20quotes.htm. Accessed September 5, 2005.

[2] Huang AJ. Rethinking the approach to beauty in medicine. Available at: http://www.jama.com. Accessed September 6, 2005.

[3] Stunkard AJ, Lafkleur WR, Wadden TA. Stigmatization of obesity in medieval times: Asia and Europe. International Journal of Obesity 1998;22: 1141–4.

[4] Spurgas AK. Body image and cultural background. Available at: http://Blackwell-synergy.com/doi/abs/10.1111/j.1475–682X.2005.00124.x?cookie Set = 1. Accessed September 6, 2005.

[5] Greenberg BS, Eastin M, Hofschire L, et al. Portrayals of overweight and obese individuals on commercial television. Am J Public Health 2003;93: 1342–8.

[6] Grizzard T. Fat bias: a barrier to the treatment of obesity. Available at: http://webweekly.hms.harvard.edu/archive/2002/9_23/student_scene.html. Accessed September 1, 2003.

[7] Balko R. The terror of fat. Available at: http://www.cato.org/cgi-bin/scripts/printtech.egi/research/articles/bal. Accessed September 21, 2005.

[8] Lundberg GD. How to prevent the obese from becoming "obeser"–stop eating. Available at: http://medscape.com/viewarticle/495270. Accessed August 26, 2005.

[9] Lundberg GD. How to prevent obesity in developed countries–part 2. Available at: http://medscape.com/viewarticle/498089. Accessed August 26, 2005.

[10] Lundberg GD. Fighting obesity–round 3. Available at: http://medscape.com/viewarticle/501950. Accessed August 26, 2005.

[11] Barclay L. Physicians not immune form anti-fat bias: a newsmaker interview with Marlene Schwartz, PhD. Available at: http://medscape.com/viewarticle/462284_print. Accessed August 13, 2005.

[12] Schwartz MB, Chambliss HO, Brownell K, et al. Weight bias among health professionals specializing in obesity. Available at: http://obesityresearch.org/cgi/content/full/11/9/1033. Accessed August 13, 2005.

[13] Chambliss HO, Finley CE, Blair S. Attitudes toward obese individuals among exercise science students. Available at: http://www.yale.edu/rudd/pdf/attitudes_towards.pdf. Accessed September 5, 2005.

[14] United Press International. Obese people neglected by some physicians. Available at: http://www.nim.nih.gov/medlineplus/news/fullstory26141.html. Accessed August 20, 2005.

[15] Weight-Control Information Network. WIN notes, research notes: physicians have negative attitudes toward obese patients. Available at: http://win.niddk.nih.gov/notes/winter04/winnotes_winter04.htm#physicians. Accessed August 13, 2005.

[16] Agency for Healthcare Research and Quality. AHRQ study finds weight-loss surgeries quadrupled in five years. Available at: http://ahrq.gov/research/jul05/0705RA23.htm. Accessed August 22, 2005.

[17] Colwell J. New ACP guidelines target obesity management. Available at: http://acponline.org/journals/news/apr05/obesity.htm. Accessed August 22, 2005.

[18] National Heart, Lung, and Blood Institute (National Institutes of Health). The practical guide: identification, evaluation, and treatment of overweight and obesity in adults. Available at: http://www.nhlbi.nih.gov/guidelines/obesity/prctgd_b.pdf. Accessed September 5, 2005.

[19] Gard M, Wright J. The obesity epidemic: science, morality, and ideology. London: Routledge; 2005.

[20] Campos P. The obesity myth: why America's obsession with weight is hazardous to your health. New York: Gotham Books, Penguin; 2004.

[21] Charon R, Montello M, editors. Stories matter: the role of narrative in medical ethics. London: Routledge; 2002.

[22] Oelschlager BK. Gastrointestinal complications of bariatric surgery. Available at: http://www.medscape.com/viewarticle/502881. Accessed August 23, 2005.

[23] The Associated Press. Woman offended by doc's obesity advice. Available at: http://news.yahoo.com/s/ap/20050824/ap_on_fe_st/obesity_complaint. Accessed August 25, 2005.

[24] ObesityHelp, Inc. WLS memorial. Available at: http://www.obesityhelp.com/morbidobesity/wlsmemorial.phtml. Accessed August 18, 2005.

ELSEVIER
SAUNDERS

Perioperative Nursing Clinics 1 (2006) 25–30

PERIOPERATIVE
NURSING
CLINICS

Developing a Business Case for Bariatric Surgery

Lorraine J. Butler, RN, BSN, MSA, CNOR

*Methodist Hospital, Clarian Health Partners, I-65 at 21st Street, P.O. Box 1367,
Room A2375, Indianapolis, IN 46206-1367, USA*

Because bariatric surgical procedures are one of the fastest growing surgical interventions both in the United States and abroad, bariatric programs require vigilant consideration before implementation. Numerous bariatric programs have failed as a result of lack of planning to ensure optimum patient outcomes and financial success.

Before a facility determines if a bariatric surgery program is appropriate for its setting, a detailed business case must be developed to ensure all actions are in the best interest of the organization. According to Schmidt [1], a business case is a tool that supports planning and decisions about whether to implement a new program, weighing the financial and other business consequences of that action. The constructive analysis documenting pros and cons of proposed initiatives of the business venture validates the benefits for consideration by senior level management. A thorough business analysis includes financial implications and provides information about existing business initiatives or processes that may be changed or influenced as a result of starting a bariatric program.

The patient population who might be seeking services in the health care setting and national averages to determine length of stay and death rate can be a baseline to determine program opportunities and financial feasibility for a health care facility. In 2002, 88% of all patients ranged between the ages of 18 and 54 years. Patients between the ages of 55 and 64 years accounted for

11% of the procedures. The >65 years age group, however, had a significant growth in bariatric surgeries. In addition, the overall length of stay decreased by 24% for all surgeries. Hospital death rates fell by 64% from 0.89% to 0.32% between 1998 and 2002. Despite this decline, the death rate for men decreased from 2.76% to 0.79%, which is three times higher than the 0.24% death rate for women (Table 1) [2,3].

Health Care Cost and Utilization Project nationwide inpatient sample 1998 to 2002

There are several driving forces required for implementing a thorough bariatric program. The first is impact on the workplace and the necessary changes. The current financial status and the ability to deliver a safe program as compared with the impact this new program will have on other facility-wide programs is a significant consideration. Another is the perception within the community and whether this program will distinguish the facility from others that do not perform bariatric surgery and the market opportunities. The financial implications require consideration of return on investment that generates the revenue stream, which may be from self-pay patients versus insurance coverage for patients. A mix of insured, partially insured, and self-pay patients can contribute to a successful program.

The last driving force is patient demand to ensure that the program remains viable because patients can and will access the services. A state-of-the art accounting and finance system that can appropriately evaluate the profit and loss for such

E-mail address: ljb038@aol.com

Table 1
National estimates of bariatric surgery use and outcomes by age and sex (1998 and 2002)

	Number of surgeries		Length-of-stay (d)		Inpatient death rate (%)	
	1998	2002	1998	2002	1998	2002
Age (y)						
12–17[a]	—	178 (31)	—	3.5 (0.3)	—	0.00 (0.00)
18–34	4336 (636)	19,554 (2202)	4.4 (0.2)	3.4 (0.1)	0.47 (0.21)	0.05 (0.04)
35–44	4825 (638)	23,404 (2667)	4.9 (0.2)	3.6 (0.1)	1.10 (0.40)	0.23 (0.07)
45–54	3320 (472)	20,264 (2124)	5.6 (0.3)	4.1 (0.2)	0.91 (0.38)	0.43 (0.11)
55–64	772 (114)	7719 (941)	5.7 (0.5)	4.3 (0.2)	0.00 (0.00)	0.93 (0.26)
65+[a]	—	615 (107)	—	6.1 (1.1)	—	1.71 (1.23)
Sex						
Male	2527 (365)	11,289 (1530)	5.9 (0.3)	4.0 (0.2)	2.76 (0.65)	0.79 (0.18)
Female	10,859 (1650)	60,444 (6976)	4.8 (0.2)	3.8 (0.1)	0.46 (0.15)	0.24 (0.05)
Total	13,386 (2021)	71,733 (8704)	4.99 (0.21)	3.80 (0.13)	0.89 (0.20)	0.32 (0.05)

Standard errors are in parentheses.

[a] The number of surgeries in age groups 12–17 and 65+ for 1998 is too small to provide a reliable estimate.

From Encinosa WE, Bernard DM, Steiner CA, et al. Use and costs of bariatric surgery and prescription weight-loss medications. Health Aff (Millwood) 2005;24(4):1039–46.

a program is a necessity. The following list[1] outlines considerations that should be included in the business plan:

- Service description with clinical and educational components
- Program objectives
- Program incentives
- Service continuum
- Technology or equipment required for the program
- Timeline (ie, length of time to increase to full incremental volume)
- Competition
- Target market and market share, including
  - Inpatient surgeries
  - Diagnosis-related groups
  - Outpatient visits
- Pricing and contracting
- Financial investment (eg, capital and operational costs), including
  - Physician full-time equivalents
  - Nonphysician full-time equivalents
  - Equipment and supplies
  - Marketing
  - Information system
  - Length and volume of operating room procedures
  - Effects on the postanesthesia care unit

- Regulatory issues
- Barriers and obstacles

Market opportunities

An external assessment of the climate and market opportunities for need, target market competition, market share or potential market share, and regulatory or legislative issues must be completed [4]. Awareness of the competition or potential competition and advertising strategies and program awareness within the community helps determine the opportunities. When awareness and opportunities need to be created for the program to start, there is an amplified need for advertising and marketing before the program begins.

Determining financial benefits

Administrative teams must make a sound commitment to execute a comprehensive program. As the financial benefits are analyzed, it is critical that competency of a referral base and surgeons are determined. A program must have a core multidisciplinary team with skills for bariatric care to benefit a program. If those skills are not present the commitment to recruit, educate, and develop the skills must be addressed before a program can be developed.

After evaluating the marketplace, the next step in the process is to meet with various insurance payors fully to understand insurance coverage

---

[1] *From* Association of periOperative Registered Nurses. AORN bariatric surgery guideline. AORN J 2004;79:1026–52; with permission.

(eg, types, rates) for bariatric procedures [5]. Many health companies stipulate that certain procedures are covered if the patient's morbid obesity has had adverse affects on the body resulting in comorbidities, which if not reversed could result in the patient's demise.

A successful bariatric program can be lucrative for the health care facility providing that the actual cost of ancillary support and labor is maintained between $7000 and $10,000 per case. Providers profiled by the Health Care Advisory Board report direct cost per case between $6500 and $11,200, reimbursement between $13,000 and $15,500, and a favorable contribution to margin [6]. These numbers indicate the typical contribution to margin per patient day is between $450 and $1750 for bariatric surgery, whereas the average contribution for all procedural cases is $898 [6].

As the total number of bariatric surgeries quadrupled from 13,386 in 1998 to 71,733 in 2002, the cost has been analyzed by the Nationwide Inpatient Sample of the Health Care Cost and Utilization Project (HCUP) for 1998 and 2002 (Table 2) [2].

The Nationwide Inpatient Sample is a database that is nationally representative of about 1000 hospitals sampled to approximate a 20% sample of United States community hospitals. Total

charges reported in the Nationwide Inpatient Sample are used with hospital-specific cost-to-cost ratios to estimate hospital costs for bariatric surgeries [2,7]. Cost-to-charge ratios are obtained from standard accounting files at the Centers for Medicare and Medicaid services. For the estimation of cost in HCUP, see Friedman and coworkers [7].

The data reveal that Medicare, Medicaid, and self-pay accounted for 6%, 5%, and 3% of bariatric surgeries, whereas 8% was by privately insured patients. In addition, nationwide facility costs for bariatric surgery increased from an estimated $157 million in 1998 to $948 million in 2002. The average cost per surgery increased by approximately 13%, from $11,705 to $13,215.

Medstat, MarketScan 2002 provided an average for bariatric surgery spending in a sample of large employers for a total of 2988 surgeries (Table 3). The total average cost for surgeries was $19,346.

Current Procedure Terminology codes are the standard for Medicare and Medicaid reimbursement and are used by many managed care and private insurance carriers. One large insurance carrier reimburses physicians at a small Philadelphia hospital approximately $1400 per case for gastric bypass for morbid obesity (Current Procedure Terminology code 43,846) [6]. Facility analysis of the profit and loss performance to

Table 2
National estimates of bariatric surgery use and costs by payer (1998 and 2002)

Payer/use and cost measure	1998	2002	Percent change (1998–2002)
Number of surgeries			
Total	13,386 (2021)	71,733 (8704)	436
Private	10,167 (1528)	59,497 (7284)	486
Medicare	1106 (209)	4261 (537)	285
Medicaid	940 (218)	3463 (615)	268
Self-pay	704 (197)	2479 (704)	252
Other	469 (192)	2033 (544)	334
Hospital costs (millions)			
Total	$157 (24)	$948 (120)	503
Private	$117 (18)	$777 (102)	564
Medicare	$15 (3)	$67 (9)	347
Medicaid	$12 (3)	$52 (13)	333
Self-pay	$8 (2)	$25 (5)	213
Mean cost per surgery			
All payers	$11,705 (578)	$13,215 (728)	12.9
Private	$11,494 (614)	$13,048 (738)	13.5
Medicare	$13,865 (1069)	$15,903 (1073)	14.6
Medicaid	$12,785 (1611)	$15,051 (2581)	17.7
Self-pay	$10,866 (1228)	$9828 (1097)	−9.6

Standard errors are in parentheses.
All costs are in 2002 US dollars and include inpatient costs only.
From Encinosa WE, Bernard DM, Steiner CA, et al. Use and costs of bariatric surgery and prescription weight-loss medications. Health Aff (Millwood) 2005;24(4):1039–46.

Table 3
Average bariatric surgery spending in a sample of large employers (2002)

Type of surgery	Number of surgeries	Average payments ($)				
		Total	Hospital	Physician	Out of pocket	Health plan
Banding and gastroplasty without bypass	117	15,704	13,320	2385	673	15,032
Gastric bypass: Roux-en-Y	2531	19,375	16,781	2595	643	18,733
Other gastric bypass[a]	276	19,914	16,566	3348	604	19,310
Revision only	64	22,387	19,293	3094	421	21,967
Total	2988	19,346	16,679	2667	635	18,710
Non-laparoscopic	2577	19,623	16,977	2646	576	19,047
Laparoscopic	411	17,608	14,813	2795	1009	16,600
Total	2988	19,346	16,679	2667	635	18,710
Without revision	2855	19,031	16,378	2653	623	18,408
With revision	133	26,105	23,134	2970	901	25,203
Total	2988	19,346	16,679	2667	635	18,710

All payments are for inpatient hospital care.
[a] Other gastric bypass includes long limb bypass and bilopancreatic diversion.
From Encinosa WE, Bernard DM, Steiner CA, et al. Use and costs of bariatric surgery and prescription weight-loss medications. Health Aff (Millwood) 2005;24(4):1039–46.

evaluate the financial soundness of a decision to start a bariatric program based on market opportunities and patient care reimbursement provides a basis for the decision to move forward.

Medstat data

Team involvement

Decisions to start the bariatric program benefit from the resources available to assess and analyze every aspect and phase of the initiative [3]. Once the external market and financial assessment establishes the opportunity, numerous roundtable discussions should be held to explore if a comprehensive bariatric program is appropriate for the facility. Using a multidisciplinary approach, the necessary services required for the continuum of care are involved in decision making. The team must determine if the health care facility's mission, vision, philosophy, and strategic plan support a bariatric program.

An internal assessment is made identifying strengths, weaknesses, opportunities, and threats if the system, as it exists, is completed. There may be current programs that will be eliminated or changes made to accommodate a start-up program for bariatric patients. These decisions influence every aspect of the functions within the health care facility.

When a facility strategizes a bariatric program they must also consider the risks and implications of such a program [8]. For example, morbidly obese patients are at a higher risk for adverse outcomes because of their comorbidities associated with their weight. These comorbidities may lead to complications because of the patient's health status. Resulting complications require further testing, treatments, possibly another surgical procedure, and increased length of stay. The multidisciplinary team may include but is not limited to:

- Administrator
- Chief financial officer or designee
- Business or marketing director
- Chief of surgery
- Chief of anesthesia
- Director of perioperative services
- Representative from patient care services
- Director of materials management

As program feasibility is established, a committee might be formed to explore clinical program needs. The clinical representatives should include, but are not limited to:

- Nutritionist
- Physical therapist
- Perioperative bariatric coordinator
- Advance nurse practitioner
- Bariatric surgeon

- Behavioral services
- Internist
- Director of radiology
- Director of gastrointestinal services

Clinical decisions might include employee education, bariatric patient programs including education and follow-up, competency assessment, equipment and supply purchases, facility changes, patient flow, and other needs. Determining preparation time is critical to plan readiness for the start of a program.

Facility changes might be necessary. Preoperative, intraoperative, and postoperative care and impact on the workplace require analysis to determine structural or procedural changes that might be required. Many facilities have created special postoperative care units, whereas some place these patients wherever a bed is available.

Availability and purchase of equipment, such as wheelchairs, stretchers, beds, toilets, lifting devices, instrumentation, operating room tables, sequential compression devices, and tourniquets, must be assessed. Specialized equipment for bariatric surgery is costly. Equipment must have the capacity to hold patients ranging up to 1000 lb. The price ranges vary depending on the vendors. In addition, a facility needs to assess the quantity of this equipment based on predicted volume and patient flow. Another avenue is rental versus purchase.

Equipment that a facility must consider for purchase should include but is not limited to that outlined in Table 4. Initially, however, equipment needs range from $30,000 bariatric beds for patient rooms to $60,000 operating room table; special anesthesia equipment; larger bariatric retractors; special titanium staples; wide wheelchairs; larger bathrooms, showers, and commodes; larger gowns; and large pulse oximeters [9].

Table 4
Estimated costs for equipment

Equipment	Estimated cost ($US)
Bariatric operating room table	30,000–60,000
Bariatric stretchers	5000–6000
Specialized instruments	15,000–20,000
Video equipment	60,000–100,000
Bariatric hospital bed	6000–10,000
Bariatric wheelchair	1000–2000
Bariatric bedside commode	500–800
Bariatric scale	1200–1500

These special needs can be extremely costly but without the proper equipment, risks are inherent. For example, if the correct size sequential compression devices are not available in adequate quantity for each and every patient undergoing bariatric and other procedures, postoperative deep vein thrombosis can develop resulting in adverse postoperative outcomes. Another example is the lack of equipment for employee use resulting in injury (ie, back injury when transferring), which is a costly outcome that can result in lack of available staff. From a financial standpoint, a goal is to minimize the cost per procedure. Supply costs vary widely from $1918 to $8509 [10]. This cost per case does not include the cost for specialized equipment to meet the needs of this patient population. Supply cost varies based on equipment and supplies requested by the surgeon. Cost per case is based on the complexity of reusable, reposable, and disposable instrumentation and can vary with use of custom kits versus other options. Contract negotiations with vendors to determine best pricing based on patient care needs are necessary to analyze the anticipated start-up and maintenance costs.

The business case varies from facility to facility. Whichever methodology is used, it is imperative to include benefits, nonbenefits, financial implications, and risks. There may be more than one option for such a program. For each option a thorough assessment must be explored and a benefit analysis devised for the major stockholders, which includes the customers and the facility. In addition, for each possible risk, a grading system must be developed. For example, a new bariatric program results in increased resource requirements that some facilities may not be able to meet. The failure of hospitals, credentialing committees, and physicians to apply consistent standards to bariatric programs has resulted in a number of surgeons with inadequate training and monitoring programs, and hospitals lacking the resources to manage morbidly obese patients [11].

Public and professional concerns about the quality of care and surgical outcomes associated with the explosive growth in bariatric surgery over the decade led to the leadership of the American Society of Bariatric Surgery to recommend the formation of an independent Surgical Review Corporation to develop and implement a program of Centers of Excellence in Bariatric Surgery to address this issue [12,13]. These centers have been noted to be optimal because they provide a comprehensive and standardized program of surgical care and long-term follow-up and management of the total care of the morbidly obese patient. Further, they were able to address the benefits, financial implications, and risks associated with such a program.

A successful bariatric program is based on a comprehensive business case that defines the scope of the bariatric program, presents various options, provides the information to make recommendations, evaluates physical and financial resources, reaches an agreement on the impact and scope of the program, and seeks senior management approval to proceed with the program. Making a difference in quality of life by helping the obese population with their choice to improve their health can be a beneficial investment with proper planning and implementation.

References

[1] Schmidt ML. The business case guide. Boston: Solution Matrix Ltd.; 1997.
[2] Healthcare Cost and Utilization Project. Databases: October 2003. Available at: http://www.hcup/us.ahrq.gov/databases, jsp. Accessed April 2, 2005.
[3] Encinosa WE, Bernard DM, Steiner CA, et al. Use and costs of bariatric surgery and prescription weight-loss medications. Health Aff (Millwood) 2005;24:1039–46.
[4] Association of periOperative Registered Nurses. AORN bariatric surgery guideline. AORN J 2004; 79:1026–52.
[5] Miller RM. Guidelines for approaching payors. Bariatrics Today 2005;2:34–5.
[6] Schoenthal A, Getzen E. Bariatric surgery and the financial reimbursement cycle. J Health Care Finance 2005;31:1–9.
[7] Friedman B, De La Mare J, Andrews R, et al. Practical options for estimating cost of hospital inpatients stays. J Health Care Finance 2002;29:1–13.
[8] Risks to consider when planning a program for bariatric Surgery. OR Manager 2003;19:10–4.
[9] Alt SJ. Market memo: bariatric surgery programs growing quickly nationwide. Health Care Strategic Management 2001;19:8.
[10] Study finds large cost variation for laparoscopic gastric bypass. OR Manager 2004;20:9–14.
[11] Steinbrook R. Surgery for severe obesity. N Engl J Med 2004;350:1075–9.
[12] Pope GB, Birkmeyer JD, Findlayson SGR. National trends in utilization and in-hospital outcomes of bariatric surgery. J Gastrointest Surg 2002;6:855–61.
[13] Liu JH, Etzioni DA, O'Connell JB, et al. Inpatient surgery in California, 1990–2000. Arch Surg 2003;138:1106–12.

ELSEVIER
SAUNDERS

Perioperative Nursing Clinics 1 (2006) 31–45

PERIOPERATIVE
NURSING
CLINICS

Weight-Loss Surgery Education for the Health Care Provider and the Weight-Loss Surgery Patient

Cheri Ackert-Burr, RN, MSN, CNOR*

US Surgical, Norwalk, CT, USA

Obesity in the United States continues to be a major concern when caring for a population where 60% of the United States is overweight and 20% to 30% is obese. That is approximately 60 million obese people in the United States, and studies show that figure is rising. The Office of the US Surgeon General reports that the risks of obesity may cause as many deaths as cigarette smoking. In January 2003, the American Medical Association stated "Obesity accounts for more than 300,000 deaths annually in the USA and will soon overtake smoking as the primary preventable cause of death if trends continue" [1]. Obesity is considered a chronic disease.

There are many special considerations and challenges that need to be addressed when caring for the weight-loss surgery patient. Education for the health care provider and for the obese patient is critical to achieve the best possible outcome not only after surgery but for the long-term success of the weight-loss surgery patient. Health care providers need to understand that obesity is a multifactorial disease. No one factor causes obesity; there are many contributing genetic, environmental, and behavioral factors (Fig. 1).

Many health care organizations have come to realize that medically managed weight loss can be successful short-term (less than 5 years), but only for a very small percentage long-term. The American Medical Association, National Institutes of Health, American Academy of Family Practitioners, and the National Institute of Diabetes and Digestive and Kidney Diseases all recognize that weight-loss surgery is the only long-term

effective treatment for obesity. The technical difficulty of the weight-loss surgery procedure demands special training for the surgeon and other members of the health care team. This article provides an overview of education needs for the different health care provider groups involved in caring for the weight-loss surgery patient. It also discusses the patient's responsibility in becoming educated about the procedure, expectations both short- and long-term, and lifestyle changes that need to be adhered to for the rest of their life.

Types of bariatric procedures

Currently, three procedures are being performed for weight-loss surgery. Each procedure offers benefits and short- and long-term challenges.

Biliopancreatic diversion with duodenal switch

The biliopancreatic diversion with duodenal switch procedure has been used since the 1960s. A sleeve resection of the stomach is completed maintaining continuity of the gastric lesser curve. The jejunum is divided and the distal limb is anastomosed to the duodenum. A jejunoileal anastomosis is formed maintaining continuity of the gastro-duodenal-jejunal axis. The food is passed into the shortened limb of the jejunum where it begins to be digested at the distal anastomosis near the ileum. This procedure is considered primarily malabsorptive (Fig. 2; Box 1).

Adjustable gastric banding

Restrictive procedures restrict the size of the stomach (Fig. 3). One of the most popular procedures is the adjustable band gastroplasty. An

* 2302 Willow Point Drive, Kingwood, TX 77339.
E-mail address: cackert-burr@hotmail.com

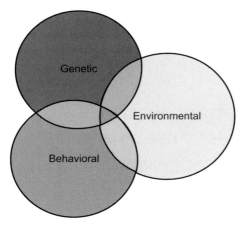

Fig. 1. Multifactorial disease. (Courtesy of US Surgical, Norwalk, CT; with permission.)

Box 1. Benefits and complications of biliopancreatic diversion with duodenal switch

Benefits
Rapid weight loss
Greater sustained weight loss with less
   dietary compliance

Complications
Increased risk of malnutrition and
   deficiency
Constant follow-up to monitor increased
   risk
Intermittent diarrhea and/or foul
   smelling stool

adjustable (ie, expandable, deflatable) band is placed around the top of the stomach, creating a pouch. This small pouch of 20 to 30 mL limits the amount of food that can be eaten at any given time. Patients must be very aware of eating healthy foods and in small amounts to have the maximum opportunity for weight loss (Box 2).

Combination procedure

The Roux-en-Y gastric bypass procedure is considered the gold standard of weight loss surgery (Fig. 4). It is primarily a restrictive

procedure; however, there is some malabsorption because of bypassing the duodenum and a portion of the proximal jejunum. A small pouch of 20 to 30 mL is made by stapling across the stomach. A Y-shaped section of the small intestine is attached to the pouch to allow food to bypass the duodenum and the first portion of the jejunum (Box 3).

Educational requirements

Caring for the weight-loss surgery patient can seem deceptively easy. Weight-loss surgery is not

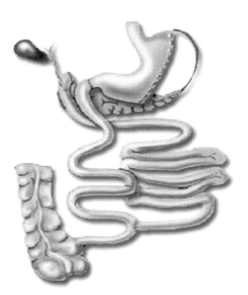

Fig. 2. Malabsorptive procedure. (Courtesy of US Surgical, Norwalk, CT; with permission.)

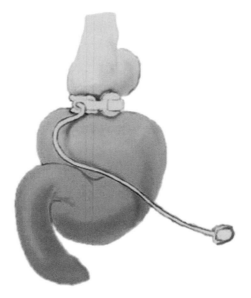

Fig. 3. Restrictive procedure. (Courtesy of US Surgical, Norwalk, CT; with permission.)

Box 2. Benefits and complications of adjustable gastric banding

Benefits
Relatively easy operation
May be safer for higher risk patients
No protein-calorie malabsorption
No vitamin or mineral deficiencies due to malabsorption

Complications
Slower weight loss
May require multiple adjustments
Risk of band erosion and band slippage
Less effective for sweet eaters
Requires significant dietary compliance

Box 3. Benefits and complications of Roux-en-Y gastric bypass procedure

Benefits
Rapid weight loss
Provides a feeling of satiety for the patient
Sustained weight loss with limited dietary compliance

Complications
Potential for leaks
Limited vitamin-B absorption
Gradual weight gain over 15 years
Vitamin and nutrient deficiencies possible

just another laparoscopic surgery. Weight-loss surgery is considered a high-risk and technically difficult procedure. For a patient to have successful outcomes there should be a comprehensive program to provide preoperative assessment screening, education, and long-term follow-up. As with any challenging program, education is of paramount importance. Each health care provider and the weight-loss surgery patient should be involved in an ongoing learning process. Each medical discipline involved in weight-loss surgery offers unique education requirements for the staff. Each type of surgical weight-loss procedure brings

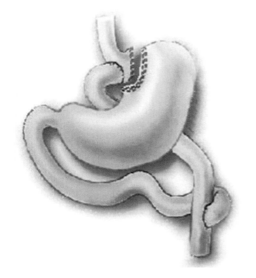

Fig. 4. Roux-en-Y gastric bypass procedure. (Courtesy of US Surgical, Norwalk, CT; with permission.)

challenges and a distinctive set of educational needs for the caregiver and the patient. Education recommendations and preparation of the health care providers and the patient are discussed at each phase of the perioperative experience.

Primary care physicians

Primary care physicians are the entry point into care for obesity control and treatment. They need to have an understanding of medically managed weight programs and weight-loss surgery options for the morbidly obese patient. Insurance companies require a medical letter of necessity from the primary care physician for the patient considering weight-loss surgery. The primary care physician not only refers eligible patients for treatment but is involved in their long-term follow-up care. They need to be cognizant of specific laboratory tests and laboratory values that are affected and other postoperative complications that can occur. Training and education for the primary care physician need to include an understanding of the areas outlined in Box 4. The primary care physician plays an important role in caring for the postsurgical weight loss patient because of the need to continue long-term medical and education follow-up.

Surgeons

The American Society for Bariatric Surgery (ASBS) strongly recommends baseline skills and learning activities for the bariatric and weight-loss surgery surgeon performing either the open or laparoscopic weight-loss procedures. The hospital

Box 4. Areas of training for the primary
care physician

Professional agencies supporting
    weight loss surgery
Physiological response to weight loss
    surgery
Resolution of comorbid conditions
Outcome data from the surgeon the
    patient is referred to
Long-term follow-up care and expected
    lab values
Diabetes: 90% of people who have
    non-insulin dependent diabetes
    mellitus are obese
Hypertension: 5–6× risk in obese
    patients
Sleep apnea: 12–30× risk
Increased cholesterol
Increased risk for myocardial infarction
Chronic venous insufficiency
Impaired immune response
Carpal tunnel syndrome
Urinary stress incontinence
Increased risk for cancer
Gout
Deep vein thrombosis
Pancreatitis
Arthritis
Joint problems
Back pain
Stroke
Cardiomyopathy
Steatohepatitis
Infertility
Chronic fatigue
Depression
Cholecystitis

includes both didactic and hands-on laboratory work involving cadavers; and

• At least three proctored cases in which the assistant is a fully trained bariatric surgeon; or
• Completion of an approved preceptorship program [3]

Outcomes should be documented for the first 15 procedures to ensure that acceptable perioperative complication rates are achieved. The facility should review the surgeon's outcome data at 6 months and on a regular basis thereafter. ASBS recommends that the surgeon participates in ongoing continuing medical education focused on the care of the bariatric patient. The surgeon also has a responsibility to participate in educational training for the health care providers and the patients.

Nursing

"Fear of the unknown causes anxiety" is one of the first things learned in nursing school about patient responses. Nowhere is that statement truer than with the nurse giving care to bariatric patients. The unknown factor, bariatric surgery, and chronic obesity it's causes, and the comorbid conditions associated with obesity lead the nurse to fear caring for a patient who he or she may believe is self-indulgent, responsible for their own condition, and could possibly cause them personal injury when mobilizing. Lack of understanding that obesity is more than calories taken in divided by expenditure results in preconceived ideas about the patient population, and can lead to misconceptions in patient care and developing a plan of care.

Although nurses have been taking care of gastric surgery patients and obese patients throughout their entire careers, the combination of the two seems to strike terror in the nurse from the preadmission phase right through the entire hospital stay. To ease the fear of the unknown, education of nursing personnel is crucial. That education includes familiarizing the caregiver with obesity, its multifactorial causes, patient sensitivity, and early recognition of postsurgery complications with each type of surgery for both short- and long-term care.

A history of bariatric surgery and its outcomes often help dispel uncertainty and give the nurse an idea of the great strides that have been made in the past few years. Often an introduction to the American Society of Bariatric Surgery and its recent efforts to establish "Centers of Excellence"

needs to have bariatric privilege requirements for open and laparoscopic procedures that specifically address training, proctoring, being proctored, training of assistants in surgery, outcomes, and continuing medical education. Active participation in bariatric continuing education is strongly recommended not only for the surgeon but also for the bariatric team [2].

ASBS recommends training for the surgeon that includes:

• Successful completion of a bariatric training course of at least 2-days duration, which for bariatric surgery sites help the nurse understand that bariatric surgery is a specialty that has a unique niche in the health care industry and is a complex program that takes much forethought and planning [4].

Having a comprehensive program for patient care is one of the keys to success for a program with acceptable outcomes. Successful programs take time and effort to establish, provide education for its many participants, and continually evaluate the effectiveness of the program. Keys to success for weight-loss surgery are compliance on the patients' part and a comprehensive program that addresses all aspects of care. Reinforcement of the program criteria at each phase of the program using ongoing assessment and intervention in the nurse's care plan provides continuity of care and decreases confusion for the health care provider and the patient. Knowledge of the program and its criteria becomes essential. The dietary changes that the patient must undergo are dramatic. The nurse must be knowledgeable of dietary guidelines and rationale to answer questions during all phases of the patient's stay. Early recognition of signs and symptoms of postsurgery complications can be life saving or help decrease the severity of the recovery regimen.

Education for the nursing staff can vary tremendously according to nursing units. All nursing units and other personnel throughout the hospital are asked to participate in patient sensitivity training because this addresses all patients who are obese or about 25% of the entire hospital patient population. Sensitivity to the obese patient is not always something that comes naturally to the nurse. Obesity is thought to be a self-based paradigm and does not always garner the same thoughtful responses that some caregivers have for the patient with other chronic diseases. These patients have been treated differently than others, often with negative connotations by health caregivers, from physicians to volunteers for years as studies have shown. Sensitivity training or actually sensitivity awareness is often enough to combat this counterproductive issue. Nursing education requirements cover a wide range of training when caring for the obese patient.

With the increase in the size of the population of the United States and an obesity rate in the 20th percentile, it is rare that at least 20% to 30% of the health care team is not obese. Every health care staff member, volunteers, and staff in administration need to understand the special needs of the obese patient. Every person should be educated to help provide a safe environment where the obese patient does not feel threatened.

Patient sensitivity awareness provides the health care worker with knowledge about what the obese person may have experienced in the past in dealing with discrimination, being the focus of ridicule, difficulty completing activities of daily living, and inappropriate treatment by health professionals. Acceptance of the patient's size, furniture that can easily accommodate extra weight and width, a patient flow that takes into account the mobility limitations of the obese patient, and sensitivity training in how to interact with the obese patient and their family are all issues that need to be addressed in a comprehensive weight-loss surgery program. Communicating the need for bariatric equipment to other health care providers, transport personnel, and volunteers provides a prepared team to assist the bariatric patient. Helping the obese patient feel safe while they are being cared for is absolutely crucial.

Preadmission and same-day-surgery unit personnel play an important part in getting the weight-loss surgery patient off to a smooth start before their procedure. A thorough nursing assessment is vitally important for referencing purposes for the postsurgery care of the patient. When a weight-loss surgery patient has complications after surgery, their condition can deteriorate very rapidly. The preoperative assessment allows the nursing staff to have a baseline assessment to evaluate postoperatively.

One of the recommendations from the ASBS is to provide a dedicated operating room team for these advanced laparoscopic procedures. The operating room team needs to understand how to care for the obese patient on a number of fronts. The weight-loss surgery procedures are technically difficult and require high levels of skill and experience using all the high-technology equipment that is required to do laparoscopic weight-loss surgery. Understanding the procedure itself plays an important part of preparing for each procedure. Each procedure brings with it special benefits and the potential for complications. Learning the specialty equipment, understanding the potential complications that can occur during the procedure, and anticipating surgeon needs are just a few of the areas for which the perioperative nurse and the operating room team must be prepared.

The operating room staff education should focus on patient safety with positioning and anesthesia as the primary focus to address the challenges caring for the obese patient. Assessing the patient preoperatively to understand mobility limitations, breathing difficulties, body shape, body mass index, and special concerns helps the perioperative nurse to design a care plan that meets the individual needs of the obese patient. Maintaining skin integrity, adequate air exchange, circulatory status, and fluid and electrolyte balance are a few of the priority nursing care needs of the obese patient.

Body shape and tissue mass present challenges that must be addressed when positioning the obese patient. Awake positioning is preferred so that the patient can respond to let the circulating nurse know if all joints and skin folds are in a neutral position. Awake positioning enables positioning based on the patient's response. Many times there is varying size in the amount of upper arm tissue compared with the forearm. The obese person requires extra padding for arms, legs, and beneath the head. Each part of the limb needs to be protected and secured during the procedure. Leg positioning can also be challenging. Protecting the ulnar nerve and the popliteal nerve are of extreme importance in the obese patient. A lumbar support may be required, particularly for patients with a pear-shaped body.

Anesthesia issues for intubation include decreased flexibility of the neck, the need to position the jaw above the chest for laryngoscope placement, and prevent loss of oxygen saturation. A rapid sequence intubation may be required because most obese persons suffer from reflux. Aspiration is a very high risk because of the low use of the lung capacity because obese patients may only use about the upper third of their lung capacity. Oxygen saturation is another concern. A thick-walled chest and underuse of the lungs can contribute rapid oxygen desaturation of the obese person.

Instrumentation is a primary area of education. The sales representatives for equipment and supplies can provide a multitude of learning modalities. Some of these include videos, step-by-step use charts, and hands-on return demonstrations. The more knowledgeable the operating room staff is about instrumentation and the procedure, the less likely the surgeon needs to divide his or her attention between the doing the procedure and teaching the staff.

Care pathways are an important part of caring for the surgical weight-loss patient because they standardize the patient care and decrease resource use without compromising outcomes [5]. Pathways provide consistency and a documented plan of care for both experienced and novice nursing staff. Having the nursing staff participate in the pathway development helps all caretakers understand what the plan of care is and how they are involved in delivering that care. Teaching the staff about pathways for the weight-loss surgery patient can be time consuming but provides a solid foundation of knowledge for that staff in the future.

Clinical nutritionist

Clinical nutrition experts play an essential role in weight-loss surgery. Special training is required, however, before the dietician begins work with weight-loss surgery patients. The weight-loss surgery patient no longer follows the traditional nutrition requirements of the food pyramid. There are physiologic responses to certain food groups that may not have been present before surgery. Clinical nutritionists need to understand that the patient no longer has the same capacity for food volume because the stomach pouch is reduced to approximately 20 to 30 mL capacity. They need to learn to prioritize food selection and timing. An example of prioritizing is getting a minimum of 75 to 80 g of protein each day. Water should not be taken with meals. It should be taken 30 minutes before eating or 30 minutes after eating. There is no longer room for both at the same time. Getting sufficient amounts of water is a struggle until the patient learns to continually sip water throughout the day. Dehydration is one of the most frequent hospital readmissions after surgery for the gastric bypass and duodenal switch patient.

Before surgery the clinical nutritionist meets with the potential patient to complete a nutritional assessment and counseling that should include eating habits, types of food, eating times, and food selection. Preoperative nutritional counseling involves behavior changes that can be expected after surgery. These include:

- Portion size
- Protein intake
- Eliminating carbonation
- Eliminating sweets or sugars
- Foods that can produce an adverse effect
- Frequency of meals
- Fluid intake
- Vitamin supplements for a lifetime

Postoperative and discharge nutritional instructions need to follow the prescribed diet that the surgeon and dietician have put together. This is based on the type of procedure, healing times for tissue, and dietary requirements to help the patient have the most successful outcome. Long-term nutritional follow-up is an integral part of the weight-loss surgery patient's continued success. Many of the patients think it is going to be easier than it is to follow the dietary requirements. The surgery is only a tool to help the obese person loose weight. Intensive dietary instruction teaches the patient how best to use that tool for optimal outcomes. Each type of procedure has different dietary requirements that not only the clinical nutritionist needs to understand but also nursing staff need to understand so that the patient receives consistent information and reinforcement of that information.

Training opportunities can be few and far between for this group of health care providers. The clinical nutritionist can participate as an allied health member with the ASBS. Networking with other experienced bariatric clinical nutritionists can help the new clinical nutritionist have a much more thorough understanding of the nutritional requirements of the weight-loss surgery patient. Practice management site visits are an excellent learning opportunity for the dietician.

Resources including nutritional presentations at the ASBS national meetings and nutritional articles in the ASBS journal are available. The American Dietetic Association offers a certification course for bariatrics weight-loss surgery. Clinical nutritionists working with weight-loss surgery patients recognize that there is minimal evidenced-based research to support what they are teaching at this time; however, laboratory values are followed very closely postoperatively to make sure that patient do not suffer vitamin and nutrient deficiencies.

Psychologist or psychiatrist

The psychologist is another vital member of the weight-loss surgery team. Most insurance companies require a preoperative psychologic assessment to determine if the patient is a candidate to undergo this surgery. Contraindications for weight-loss surgery include:

- High-risk medical patient (super morbidly obese)
- Unable to understand the procedure
- Unrealistic expectations

- Unresolved emotional illness
- Drug abuse or alcoholism
- Unmanaged or out of control comorbid conditions
- Women who are thinking about becoming pregnant in the near future

Behavior modification increases the chances of the weight-loss surgery patient continuing to be successful in their weight loss and maintaining that weight loss. The patient needs to learn about changing their eating habits. Part of the assessment focuses on how they eat (grazing, sweet eater, binge eater, or yo-yo dieter). The person who uses food as a coping mechanism for stress, anger, happiness, and as a substitute for attention needs to understand why they eat the way they do. Emotional eating continues to be a challenge.

Education and training for the psychologist needs to build on already existing professional information. The psychologist working with the weight-loss surgery patient population needs to understand not only the behavior changes needed for the weight-loss surgery patient to continue to be successful, but also to have a thorough understanding of how the surgical procedure affects the patient physiologically postoperatively. The psychologist continues to be an integral part of the weight-loss surgery team. Educational opportunities for the psychologist include articles from their professional organization, ASBS affiliation, and practice management site visits with established weight-loss programs. Support groups for the weight-loss surgery patient provide the psychologist with a regular opportunity to interact with the patients in a group forum and to meet selectively for one-on-one counseling.

The psychologist plays a key role in the follow-up care of the weight-loss surgery patient. Helping the patient to understand physical changes, emotional changes, and how to deal with life changes after surgery can provide the post–weight-loss surgery patient with ongoing support and an opportunity for continued success.

Patient education

The importance of patient education has been proved time and again. AORN standards [2] suggest using knowledge deficit as a major component of the care plan. This involves all departments that interact with the patient during their hospitalization. Every department needs to develop a pathway for this patient that addresses education and patient care needs.

There are many facets of patient education for the weight-loss surgery patient. This is one of the most informed patient populations in the health care setting today. Many of these patients started their education process by talking with other patients who have undergone the weight-loss surgery and have been successful. Active participation by the patient in activities before surgery increases the likelihood of a successful outcome. Preoperatively there are many areas that the interested consumer can research for information.

Most programs have very extensive patient education protocols. The potential patient is required to attend a patient education seminar usually presented by the surgeon and the hospital or office bariatric coordinator. This can be a power point presentation, a patient education video, or patient education literature and may include a patient surgery test, which documents the patient's understanding of the procedure and what is expected. Other information avenues include web sites for obesity and local and regional hospital web sites. The patient should be encouraged to attend more than one patient education program to determine if the program meets their needs. The patient should feel comfortable with the surgeon and the bariatric team because this is a long-term relationship. Weight-

loss surgery patients must be educated because they are very involved in the decision-making process not only to have surgery but in choosing the procedure that best fits their needs.

Another important issue for the patient to understand is that weight-loss surgery is not a cure for obesity. It is only a tool and can only be successful if the patient is willing to follow the health regimen after the surgery. Most patient education focuses on behavior changes that primarily include eating habits and dietary changes. The patient needs to understand the importance of listening to their body's response to food. Responses to food triggers vary with the patient and the type of procedure that they had performed. Sweets, carbonated beverages, flour-based products, certain types of meats, and simple carbohydrates, not chewing food completely, and eating too fast present multiple challenges and responses from the body. Dumping syndrome, nausea, vomiting, diarrhea, and foul-smelling gas can be negative reinforcement for not following the prescribed diet.

Preoperatively, the patient needs access to the program requirements to see if they are an eligible candidate for the surgery. This involves completing an information intake form. They are asked for their height and weight. This allows the first

Table 1
Changes in comorbidity after laparoscopic Roux-en-Y gastric bypass

Comorbidity	Total	Aggravated (%)	Unchanged (%)	Improved (%)	Resolved (%)
Osteoarthritis/degenerative joint disease	64	2	10	47	41
Hypercholesterolemia	62	0	4	33	63
Gastroesophogeal reflux disorder	58	0	4	24	72
Hypertension	57	0	12	18	70
Sleep apnea	44	2	5	19	74
Hypertriglyceridemia	43	0	14	29	57
Depression	36	8	37	47	8
Peripheral edema	31	0	4	55	41
Urinary incontinence	18	0	11	39	44
Asthma	18	6	12	69	13
Diabetes	18	0	0	18	82
Migraine headaches	7	0	14	29	57
Anxiety	7	0	50	17	33
Venous insufficiency	7	0	71	29	0
Gout	7	0	14	14	72
Coronary heart disease	6	0	0	75	26
Chronic obstructive pulmonary disease	3	0	33	67	0
Congestive heart failure	3	0	33	67	0
Obesity hyperventilation syndrome	2	0	0	50	50

From Schauer PR, Ikramuddin S, Gourash W, et al. Outcomes after laparoscopic Roux-en-Y bypass for morbid obesity. Ann Surg 2000;232(4):515–29; with permission.

contact person to calculate their body mass index. The patient needs to meet National Institutes of Health criteria: a body mass index greater than 40 or a body mass index 35 to 40 with at least two significant comorbid conditions. This is usually about 100 lb over ideal body weight for men and 80 lb for women.

Insurance coverage is the next hurdle. Many insurance companies require very specific consultations and a medically managed weight program for a specified amount of time. It is the patient's responsibility to make sure that their insurance covers the procedure. If it does not, then the patient needs to decide if they would like to pursue the surgery without insurance coverage, or as a self-paying patient.

Once the patient has committed to the decision to have surgery, there are many preoperative learning opportunities that the patient is required to attend. Most programs require the obese patient to attend a minimum of one patient education information session that thoroughly describes the insurance precertification requirements, medical consults that may be required, different surgical procedures available in the

program, the benefits, and the possible complications of each procedure. Long-term life and behavior changes are also discussed. Most programs have the psychologist do a portion of the presentation and there is a presentation from the dietician. Preoperative instructions should include:

- Nothing by mouth status; no "last supper syndrome"
- Surgical site skin preparation
- What to wear and bring to the hospital
- Stop oral contraceptives 1 month before surgery and substitute at least two others
- Medication changes
- Diet instructions postsurgery
- Pain management
- Expected activity and ambulation postsurgery

There are patients who exhibit lack of recall, understanding, and knowledge that was shared before surgery during the postoperative phases, despite the preoperative emphasis [6]. For this reason, it is important adequately to assess the level of knowledge postoperative and reinforce and continue immediately postoperative (eg, as soon

---

Box 5. Resources on the Web

- American Association of Critical-Care Nurses (http://www.aacn.org)
- American Heart Association (http://www.americanheart.org)
- Association of periOperative Registered Nurses (http://www.aorn.org)
- American Society for Bariatric Surgery (http://www.asbs.org)
- DietWatch: nutritional information (http://www.dietwatch.com)
- American Dietetic Association (http://www.eatright.org/adap0197.html)
- American College of Surgeons (http://www.facs.org)
- Hospital and Health Networks (http://www.hhnmag.com)
- Joint Commission on Patient Safety (http://www.jcpatientsafety.org)
- Medline Education (http://www.medline.com)
- Medscape Education (http://www.medscape.com)
- State Insurance Commissions on the Web (http://www.members.tripod.com/proagency/insurance3.html)
- American Obesity Association (http://www.obesity.org)
- ObesityHelp, Inc. (http://www.obesityhelp.com)
- The International Federation for the Surgery of Obesity (http://www.obesity-online.com)
- Obesity Meds and Research New (http://www.obesity-news.com)
- Obesity Surgery Including Laparoscopy and Allied Care (http://www.obesitysurgery.com)
- Psychosomatic Medicine (http://www.psychosomaticmedicine.org)
- American Obesity Association (http://www.shapeup.org/publicaitons/guide2/app2.pdf)
- National Institutes of Health (http://text.nlm.hih.gov/nih/cdc/www/84txt.html)
- World Health Organization: Obesity—Preventing and Managing the Global Epidemic (http://www.who.int/dsa/justpub/justpub.htm#Obesity)

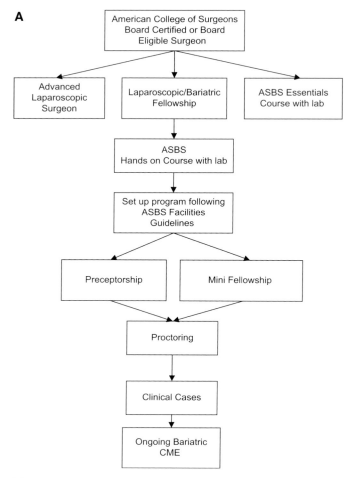

Fig. 5. (*A*) Surgeon training pathway. (*B*) Perioperative weight-loss surgery pathway. (*C*) Patient education pathway. (*D*) Bariatric education pathway. (*E*) Patient care pathway template. ASBS, American Society for Bariatric Surgery; CEO, Chief Executive Officer; CFO, Chief Financial Officer; CME, Continuing Medical Education; COO, Chief Operating Officer; OR, operating room; OT, occupational therapist; PCT, patient care technician; PT, physical therapist; RN, registered nurse; RT, respiratory therapist.

as they are admitted to the SICU, bariatric nursing unit). Pain management, ambulation, dietary regime, inspirometry, sequential compression devices, and wound care and skin care are the focus of education immediately postoperatively. The information is supplemented each day to prevent immediate education overload. Opportunities for this education should be presented on several different fronts: television videos on the patient education channel; prepared booklets from the bariatric coordinator; the diet program, which should address postoperative Days 1 and 2, and day of discharge; and information from physical therapy. The patient may need to have special

learning needs addressed in the same manner as the health care team.

Discharge education for the patient should include signs and symptoms of complications to a degree that they understand when to return to the emergency department or when to call the surgeon or bariatric coordinator. Explanations of acceptable activity levels including exercise, first postoperative office visit, and dietary progression should be discussed. All instructions should be given verbally and in written form. Most discharge education should be at a fifth grade reading level. It is important to remember that there may be a need to print the material in other

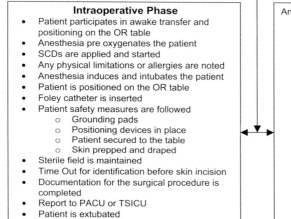

Preoperative Phase

- Patient arrives to Same Day Surgery Unit
- Chart completed by RN
- Lovenox administered
- Patient identified by Operating Room Nurse
- Bariatric bed may be ordered for each patient if patient's weight is > 350 pounds
- IV may or may not be started in Same Day Surgery or Holding Area
- Patient brought to the room by anesthesia
- OR nurse to check for Bariatric bed if it is ordered

Intraoperative Phase

- Patient participates in awake transfer and positioning on the OR table
- Anesthesia pre oxygenates the patient
- SCDs are applied and started
- Any physical limitations or allergies are noted
- Anesthesia induces and intubates the patient
- Patient is positioned on the OR table
- Foley catheter is inserted
- Patient safety measures are followed
  - Grounding pads
  - Positioning devices in place
  - Patient secured to the table
  - Skin prepped and draped
- Sterile field is maintained
- Time Out for identification before skin incision
- Documentation for the surgical procedure is completed
- Report to PACU or TSICU
- Patient is extubated
- Positioning devices and SCDs go with the patient

Anesthesia

- Identifies patient
- Starts IV in Same Day Surgery or Holding Area or OR room
- Transports patient to the room
- Assists in transferring the patient to the OR table
- Medications are given
- Rapid sequence intubation is done
- I & O monitored
- Balanced anesthesia is utilized during the procedure
- Patient is awakened post surgery
- Patient is extubated
- Patient is transferred to the Bariatric Bed
- Patient is transported to PACU or TSICU

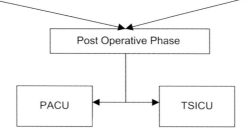

Post Operative Phase

PACU   TSICU

Fig. 5 (*continued*)

languages to facilitate learning and compliance. The health care provider discharging the patient needs to make certain that the patient clearly understands the discharge and follow-up instructions. There should be a document trail of all patient education that has taken place.

Weight-loss surgery patients need reinforcement and long-term follow-up with education. One of the best ways to accomplish this is during a regular support group meeting. Support groups allow the surgeon, bariatric coordinator, clinical nutritionist, and psychologist a venue to continue the education process. Usually the support group

meetings are held once a month. The first part of the meeting is for educational purposes followed by breakout sessions. Breakout sessions offer an opportunity for the postsurgery patients to meet and discuss changes that occur in their body and what to expect after surgery. Different issues arise as the patient progresses along the health continuum, but similarities are seen among patients at each stage in the process. The support group should be facilitated by a health care professional so that patients sharing information do not share incorrect information and a qualified person can address any clinical issues. Support

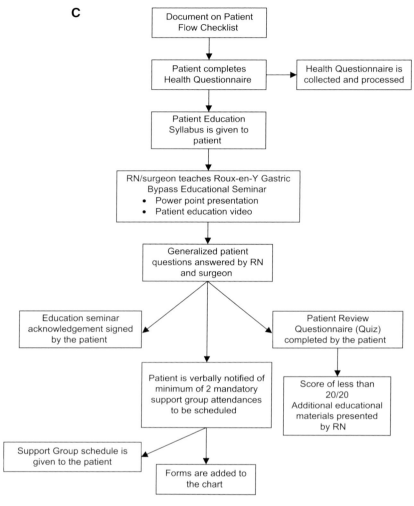

Fig. 5 (*continued*)

group topics can provide ongoing education opportunities and allow patients to participate in learning more about themselves and others in their group.

Long-term follow-up

One of the historical problems with weight-loss surgery has been the outcomes tracking data. ASBS has chosen to address this issue by requiring Centers of Excellence in Bariatric Surgery to maintain and follow postsurgery patients for a minimum of 5 years. The ASBS has indicated that this gives a much clearer picture of how successful the patients are with keeping the weight off and allows the surgeon to document complication rates and comorbid condition status changes over that period of time (Table 1). Weight loss is the primary reason patients undergo weight-loss surgery. The long-term benefit of weight-loss surgery is the resolution or improvement of comorbid conditions. The patient needs to be monitored closely to determine vitamin and nutrient deficiencies. Most weight-loss surgery patients need to take a daily multivitamin, vitamin B_{12}, and calcium citrate for the rest of their lives. Other supplements may be added as needed. The surgeon and primary care physician need to work together with the patient after surgery to provide long-term follow-up care.

D

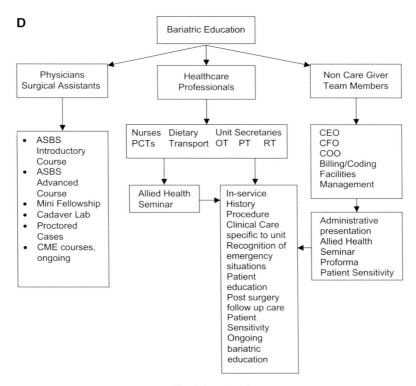

Fig. 5 (*continued*)

Strategies for learning

Adults learn in different ways. Some can read anything and understand, whereas another person does much better if they hear a verbal presentation. Some skill sets require demonstration and then a return demonstration, such as employees learning equipment use. It presents a challenge for the educator to provide a comprehensive bariatric training program.

There are a wide variety of teaching and learning opportunities for the educator to use in a variety of ways. A good starting point is to formulate a plan to provide opportunities for the staff that not only meet their learning needs but can be presented in the medium that allows them to retain best what is presented. A combination of learning activities works well. Some of the issues dealt with in formulating a plan include number of people on a shift, designated inservice times, levels of education, job responsibilities, literacy level, language barriers, motivation to learn, and staff attitude toward a subject they may not embrace.

Helpful tools are available including numerous web sites with information (Box 5). In the

everincreasing high-technology environment, the educator needs to use that to their advantage. Power point presentations can be put on compact disks with speaker notes that are visible for the participant. A 10-question test can be placed at the end of the presentation to provide evidence of learner participation. The Association of Perioperative Registered Nurses journal has several home study continuing education articles that can be used for another type of self-study project. Each of these articles has a postactivity test that can be used for documentation of participation or can be returned to AORN for continuing education credit. The American Association of Critical Care Nurse's journal has published several articles on pulmonary embolism, deep vein thrombosis, and care of weight-loss surgery patients. Some of these articles have postactivity tests and can be turned in for continuing education credit. Medscape and Medline offer articles that can be used as self-study projects. Another gold mine for educational opportunities is to request that sales representatives provide inservices on supplies and equipment that address care of the obese

E

Activity	Preadmission Office	OP Day Preoperative	OP Day Intraoperative	OP Day Postoperative
Tests				
Medications				
Diet				
Patient Education				
Attending Physician Assessment				
Attending Physician Procedure				
Nursing Assessment				
Nursing Procedures				
Consults				
Patient Activity				
Expected Outcomes				
Other				

Fig. 5 (*continued*)

patient. Many of the sales representatives provide additional programs associated with bariatrics, such as wound management, mobilizing the obese patient, recognizing postoperative complications in the weight-loss surgery patient, reconditioning of the obese patient for exercise activity, and nutritional requirements for the weight-loss surgery patient. Competency testing and story boards offer another visual learning opportunity. Off shift and weekend staff may require creative learning strategies so that they too understand the fragile nature of the obese patient and are equipped to meet their special needs.

The nurse and other team members involved in patient education need to remember that the education instructions must be presented in a variety of ways. The patient education needs to be validated for understanding. Each patient learning activity needs to be carefully documented.

Summary

Educating health care providers, patients, and the community about weight-loss surgery helps people better understand the scope of doing surgery to help people loose weight. Knowledge of weight-loss surgery and all that it involves is critical to the health care team. Meeting the educational needs of the weight-loss surgery patient and the health care provider can be challenging. Pathways and care plans can provide a firm foundation for putting together an educational program (Fig. 5). Once the program has been developed the team needs continually to update their education information. As research on this topic continues, weight-loss surgery programs will have evidence-based information to use to improve their patient care and follow-up routines.

Further readings

Alspach G. Caring for preceptors: a survey of what they need and want in educational support. Critical Care Nurse 2005;25:8–11.

Alspach G. Communicating health information an epidemic of the incomprehensible. Critical Care Nurse 2004;24:8–13.

Andrus S, Dubois J, Jansen C, et al. Teaching documentation tool: building a successful discharge. Critical Care Nurse 2003;23:39–48.

Association of periOperative Registered Nurses (AORN). Clinical path template. In: 2005 Standards, recommended practices, and guidelines. Denver (CO): AORN, Inc.; 2005. p. 103–11.

Association of periOperative Registered Nurses (AORN). Statement on the role of the health care industry representative in the operating room. In: 2005 Standards, recommended practices, and guidelines. Denver (CO): AORN, Inc.; 2005. p. 28–9.

Barone CP, Pablo CS, Barone GW. Postanesthetic care in the critical care unit. Critical Care Nurse 2004;24: 38–45.

Charlebois D, Wilmoth D. Critical care of patients with obesity. Critical Care Nurse 2004;24:19–27.

Dreger V, Tremback T. Optimize patient health by treating literacy and language barriers. AORN Journal 2002;75:278–304.

Endinosa WE, Bernard DM, Steiner CA, et al. Trends: use and costs of bariatric surgery and prescription weight-loss medications. Health Aff (Millwood) 2005;24:1039–46.

Flancbaum L. The doctor's guide to weight loss surgery, how to make the decision that could save your life. New York: Bantam Books; 2003.

Ferraro DR. Laparoscopic adjustable gastric banding for morbid obesity. AORN Journal 2003;77:923–44.

Graling P, Elariny H. Perioperative care of the patient with morbid obesity. AORN Journal 2003;77: 801–24.

Hand E. Surviving clinical competencies: taking the immunity challenge. Critical Care Nurse 2002;22(1): 87–8.

Joint Commission International Center for Patient Safety. Speak up: new education campaign offers patients tips for continuing recovery after leaving the hospital. Available at: http://www.jcipatientsafety. org. Accessed September 2005.

Lucas A. Competency program accommodates mix of nursing needs. Critical Care Nurse 2005;25:71–2.

Maiocco G. Posters give nursing staff consistent information. Critical Care Nurse 2002;22:152.

McCall JA. Progressive critical care education. Critical Care Nurse 2002;22(4):87–8.

North American Association for the Study of Obesity. 2000 Annual Meeting. Available at: http://www. naaso.org. Accessed September 2005.

Toby Haghenbeck K. Follow the rules to safer care delivery. Critical Care Nurse 2003;23:69–71.

References

[1] American Medical Association. Roadmaps for clinical practice, case studies in disease prevention and health promotion, assessment and management of adult obesity: a primer for physicians, introduction and clinical considerations (2003). Available at: http://www. ama-assn.org/ama1/upload/mm/433/booklet1.pdf.

[2] Association of periOperative Registered Nurses (AORN). AORN bariatric surgery guideline. In: 2005 Standards, recommended practices, and guidelines. Denver (CO): AORN, Inc.; 2005. p. 55–73.

[3] American Society for Bariatric Surgery (ASBS). Guidelines for granting privileges in bariatric surgery. Obesity Surgery 2003;13:238–40.

[4] Surgical Review Corporation. Centers of excellence. Available at: http://www.surgicalreview.org/about_us. html. Accessed October 2005.

[5] Yeats M, Wedergren S, Fox N, et al. The use and modification of clinical pathways to achieve specific outcomes in bariatric surgery. Am Surg 2005;71: 152–4.

[6] Madan AK, Tichansky DS. Patients postoperatively forget aspects of preoperative patient education. Obes Surg 2005;15:1066–9.

ELSEVIER
SAUNDERS

Perioperative Nursing Clinics 1 (2006) 47–53

PERIOPERATIVE
NURSING
CLINICS

Patient Preparation and Education: Bariatric Surgery

Denise O'Brien, MSN, APRN,BC, FAAN[a],*, William C. Palazzolo, MS, PA-C[b]

[a]*Department of Operating Rooms/PACU, University of Michigan Hospitals and Health Centers, UH 1C206K, 1500 Medical Center Drive, Ann Arbor, MI 48109–0044, USA*
[b]*Bariatric Surgery, University of Michigan Hospitals and Health Centers, Ann Arbor, MI, USA*

The latest data from the National Center for Health Statistics show that 30% of United States adults 20 years of age and older (over 60 million people) are obese, and this number continues to rise. This increase is not limited to adults. The percentage of young people who are overweight has more than tripled since 1980. Among children and teenagers aged 6 to 19 years, 16% (over 9 million young people) are considered overweight [1].

When other therapies (ie, dietary therapy, physical activity, behavior therapy, combined therapy, pharmacotherapy) fail to reduce weight, patients turn to surgical treatment (weight-loss surgery) [2]. Benefits of surgical treatment include durable weight loss; resolution of type 2 diabetes; lower risk of premature death; improved quality of life; lower disability and health care costs; and improvement in hypertension, cardiovascular status, obstructive sleep apnea, and benign intracranial hypertension [3].

In the next few years, bariatric surgery will be performed in every major American hospital [4]. Appropriate patient selection and preparation are keys to successful bariatric surgery outcomes. This article focuses on preparing the patient for bariatric surgery, including patient selection, preoperative testing, and education.

Patient selection criteria

As Brolin [5] states, patients undergoing bariatric procedures need to "be selected with rigor and caution." Not all persons who are obese are candidates for weight-loss surgery. Bariatric surgery programs have established patient selection criteria based on recommendations of the National Institutes of Health and the American Society for Bariatric Surgery [2,6]. Patient selection criteria are summarized in Box 1 [5–8].

Patients need to be carefully screened for bariatric surgery and operative risk established. Unacceptable operative risks include patients with unstable or severe coronary artery disease, severe pulmonary disease, and other conditions that may compromise anesthesia management or wound healing [9]. Patients who suffer from a history of alcohol dependency, drug abuse, eating disorders, or other psychologic disorders may be poor candidates for weight-loss procedures [3,10]. Contraindications may also include active peptic ulcer, hiatal hernia, inflammatory gastrointestinal disorders, or previous abdominal surgery [10].

Reliable contraception is necessary during the preparation phase and following the operative procedure. Women who are pregnant or plan to become pregnant within 12 to 24 months after surgery are not candidates for surgery (Box 2) [3,11].

Patient preparation process

The preparation of the patient for weight-loss surgery is lengthy. The patient needs to be well informed, motivated, and willing to participate in the preoperative and postoperative process. The process includes dietary counseling and lifestyle changes. A multidisciplinary team including physicians, nurses, physician assistants, dieticians, psychologists, and other specialists evaluate patients for inclusion in the program.

---

* Corresponding author.
E-mail address: dedeo@umich.edu (D. O'Brien).

1556-7931/06/$ - see front matter © 2006 Elsevier Inc. All rights reserved.
doi:10.1016/j.cpen.2005.12.003

Box 1. Patient selection criteria

Body mass index >40 or >35 with
   a serious obesity-related comorbidity
Documented unsuccessful weight loss
   attempts
Age 18 to 60 (adolescents and patients
   in their 70s may be candidates)
Absence of endocrine disorders that
   can cause massive obesity
Acceptable operative risks
Psychologically sound
Commitment to postoperative follow-up

_____

(*Data from* Refs. [5–8].)

Initial contact with the patient may be through a call center or referral. Program information and selection criteria enable the patient an opportunity to evaluate whether he or she may be eligible for weight-loss surgery. At the University of Michigan Health System, first steps include attending an information session that outlines the program requirements (see Box 2) and process for potential candidates. All programs need to include information on types of surgical procedures available for weight loss, the anatomy involved, rationale and goals for surgery, the risks and potential complications of the various surgical procedures, dietary and lifestyle modifications, anticipated outcomes, and the long-term effects of surgery [12].

Following attendance at an informational session, the patient begins the evaluation process with medical record review and psychologic and nutritional screening. When the screening is complete, the bariatric surgery team reviews the information from the evaluation process and recommendations are made. Nutritional counseling by a registered dietician is started with education on dietary changes, avoidance of nutritional complications including protein malnutrition, vitamin and mineral deficiencies, and postoperative dietary changes. The intent is to encourage the patient to lose minimally 15 pounds to decrease liver size and to incorporate healthy eating habits.

When the patient has lost the necessary weight and has completed counseling, he or she meets with the surgeon to prepare for the surgical procedure. At this time, the history and physical is completed, questions answered, operative consent signed, additional testing obtained, and the surgery date is scheduled.

Preanesthesia evaluation by an anesthesia clinician should occur minimally 1 day before, and when possible 1 month before, the scheduled weight-loss surgery [13]. Extended preanesthesia assessment may be needed if the patient has comorbidities that require evaluation. The American Society of Anesthesiologists has published guidelines for preanesthesia evaluation of patients undergoing surgery [14].

Preoperative assessment and testing

The overall goal of preoperative assessment and testing is to evaluate the patient for the weight-loss surgery and to optimize the patient for the surgical procedure. The assessments include behavioral and psychologic evaluation, laboratory and diagnostic testing, and evaluation of comorbities that may increase the patient's operative risk.

Behavioral and psychologic evaluation by a credentialed expert in psychology and behavior change identifies contraindications to weight-loss surgery [8]. An Ad Hoc Behavioral Health Committee of the Allied Health Sciences Section of the American Society for Bariatric Surgery has published suggestions for the presurgical psychologic assessment of patients anticipating weight-loss surgery [15]. Behavioral assessment includes previous attempts at weight management, eating and dietary styles, physical activity and inactivity, substance use, health-related risk-taking behavior, and legal history. Cognitive and emotional assessment include cognitive functioning; knowledge of morbid obesity and surgical interventions; coping skills, emotional modulation, and boundaries; psychopathology; and developmental history, current life situation, motivation, and expectations. Psychologic testing using standardized tests includes multiscale, single-scale, and specialized inventories. Multiscale inventories assess different aspects of a person's emotional functioning or personality based on responses to a set of questions. Shorter single-scale inventories assess a specific emotional problem, such as depression or anxiety. Specialized inventories measure quality of life or measure eating behavior.

Preanesthesia laboratory and diagnostic testing may include complete blood count, chemistry screen, iron-iron binding, vitamin B_{12}, urinalysis, blood typing, chest radiograph, and electrocardiogram. Fifteen percent to 25% of morbidly obese

---

Box 2. University of Michigan Health System patient criteria

All patients must meet the criteria outlined below to be considered a candidate for the University of Michigan Health System Bariatric Surgery Program. Please carefully review the criteria before registering.

Must be between 18 and 60 years of age. Requests for patients between 61 and 65 years require approval by bariatric surgery director and medical director.

Body mass index of 40 or greater, or 35 with life-threatening comorbidities (hypertension, heart disease, diabetes, pulmonary hypertension, sleep apnea, hyperlipidemia, polyarthritis).

Documented compliance with an unsuccessful medically supervised weight-loss program for a minimum of 6 months with monthly visits documenting weight, diet, exercise, and lifestyle modifications within the past 2 years. (Note: This may vary based on individual health insurance carrier's requirements.)

Medical evaluation and documented work-up to rule out underlying treatable causes for morbid obesity within the past year.

Psychologic evaluation must be done by a qualified mental health provider, knowledgeable in bariatric surgery, within 6 to 12 months of the appointment with the surgeon.

Must attend at least one University of Michigan Health System bariatric surgery program gastric bypass information session. This must be attended before enrolling in the program.

Weight-loss surgery is not to be performed in the presence of certain medical and psychologic diagnoses. The following are absolute contraindications:
Pregnancy, lactation
Active substance abuse
End-stage cardiovascular disease
Severe or uncontrolled psychiatric disorders
Anorexia

Relative contraindications for surgery include the following:
Unstable medical condition
Kidney disease
Active binge eating disorder or bulimia nervosa

---

patients suffer from cholelithiasis [5]. Patients with clinical symptoms of cholelithiasis undergo an abdominal ultrasound or CT for evaluation. Screening for *Helicobacter pylori* should be done and, if present, treated before surgery. Minimum laboratory testing includes liver function tests, hematocrit, glucose, creatinine, and blood urea nitrogen within 6 months of the scheduled surgical procedure [13].

Comorbidities include obstructive sleep apnea, cardiovascular disease, liver disease, and history of smoking, or difficult venous or arterial access related to obesity. Ideally, the assessment occurs before the day of surgery and the patient optimized for surgery during the waiting period before the scheduled procedure.

Obstructive sleep apnea occurs frequently in the obese patient population. Signs and symptoms include cessation of airflow for greater than 10 seconds five or more times per hour of sleep and usually associated with an oxygen saturation decrease of >4%, increased neck circumference, snoring, daytime sleepiness, or fatigue [8,16]. Patients should be screened for sleep apnea and referred for sleep evaluation when appropriate. Treatment should begin before surgery is scheduled. Compliance with continuous positive airway pressure or bilevel positive airway pressure may be greater postoperatively if patients have an opportunity to become accustomed to the devices before surgery [17]. Patients are instructed to bring their fitted masks from home on the day of surgery.

The laboratory and diagnostic testing may identify cardiovascular disease or increased risk of cardiovascular disease. Abir and Bell [18] state that "clinically severe obesity is associated with a higher frequency of cardiovascular disease, including essential hypertension, pulmonary hypertension, left ventricular hypertrophy, congestive heart failure, and ischemic heart disease." Patients with known cardiovascular disease should receive perioperative β-blockers to reduce cardiovascular complications [8]. Guidelines from the American College of Cardiology and American Heart Association recommend perioperative β-blockers for patients with coronary artery disease or two or more risk factors for coronary artery disease unless contraindicated [19].

Laboratory testing may indicate need for evaluation of hepatic function. Liver disease including fatty liver disease, cirrhosis, fibrosis, or hepatic dysfunction may necessitate intraoperative liver biopsy and further evaluation [8].

Patients who smoke increase their risk for postoperative respiratory complications [20]. Smoking cessation should be encouraged for patients who smoke cigarettes at least 6 to 8 weeks before surgery. Nicotine replacement or pharmacologic therapy (bupropion) may help reduce withdrawal symptoms and minimize risk of weight gain [8].

Peripheral and central venous access sites should be evaluated before the day of surgery. If difficult access is anticipated or the patient requires invasive monitoring, the anesthesia care provider should discuss this with the patient at that time [21].

Other issues that need to be addressed during the preoperative period include facility preparation. Bariatric equipment and supplies must be available to provide safe and dignified care for the weight-loss surgery patient.

Patient education

The patient preparing for weight-loss surgery begins his or her education during the initial phases of the program. During this time, extensive nutritional and lifestyle change education are provided. As the surgery date approaches, education focuses more specifically on perioperative care.

Preoperative education provides the patient, family, and companions with information to prepare them for the weight-loss surgery, from initial preparation to the day of surgery to follow-up care. Preparation through education improves compliance, decreases length of stay, and reduces anxiety. Evidence supporting adequate patient education and its benefits across multiple patient populations and age groups spans nearly 50 years.

Breenhaar and coworkers [22], Lithner and Zilling [23], and Garretson [24] summarize this evidence in articles on patient education and preparation programs.

Patient education during the preoperative phase of care focuses on general perioperative information and information specific to the patient's assessed needs and operative procedure. General information includes patient arrival at the facility, where to go, who and what to bring, and usual care before and after surgery. It is important for the patient's support structure (ie, spouse, family, friends) to be well informed of all the potential lifelong changes the patient will undergo. The goal is to provide a supportive environment so the patient's adjustment postoperatively is as smooth as possible. Family and friends can help in the adjustment process.

For patients undergoing weight-loss surgery, patient education includes discussion of general anesthesia with endotracheal intubation, placement of a Foley catheter and nasogastric tube, and immediate postanesthesia care. The patient may be observed in the ICU overnight or may go from the postanesthesia care unit directly to a general surgical unit. Length of postoperative stay varies with procedure and approach, averaging 2 days with laparoscopic approaches and 5 days with open procedures. Patients are expected to be out of bed the day of surgery and up ambulating on the day of surgery. Diet is nothing by mouth on the day of surgery, progressing to ice chips and clear liquids on postoperative Day 1. Patients using medications need to be instructed not to take whole pills for the first 4 weeks postoperatively [5]. Medications are either crushed if possible or provided as an elixir.

Lifelong requirements for diet and lifestyle include eating small portions of a high-protein, low-fat, low-carbohydrate diet; avoidance of sweets, alcohol, and caffeine; regular physical activity; daily vitamin and mineral supplementation; and follow-up care [7]. It is crucial the patient regularly follows-up with the bariatric team. Postoperative visits are scheduled at 2 weeks, 2 months, 6 months, 12 months, and then annually. At these visits, the patient is assessed for weight loss and complications, wounds checked, diets adjusted and monitored, and laboratories drawn to screen for vitamin-mineral-protein deficiencies.

Education related to postoperative comfort and pain management should be included in the preoperative educational plan. Depending on the type of procedure (laparoscopic or open), pain may be managed using patient-controlled analgesia or epidural analgesia. Patients need information and instructions on use of these analgesic techniques before the day of surgery and to have the techniques reviewed on the day of surgery. Discussion regarding self-reporting of pain intensity should also occur preoperatively and the appropriate pain intensity scale determined. Additional information and education related to pain and comfort management can be found in the American Society of PeriAnesthesia Nurses Acute Pain and Comfort Clinical Guideline, available from http://www.aspan.org/PDFfiles/pain&comfort.pdf.

Patients who use continuous positive airway pressure or bilevel positive airway pressure for management of their obstructive sleep apnea should be instructed to bring specially fitted masks or devices on the day of surgery. Institutional policies vary and define whether patients should bring their own equipment or if the facility provides the necessary devices for postoperative airway management of obstructive sleep apnea. Continuous oxygen saturation monitoring using pulse oximetry is recommended for the postoperative care of patients with a history of obstructive sleep apnea (Box 3) [25,26].

Day of surgery

Care of the patient and family or companions on the day of surgery should focus on emotional support and final preparation for the surgical procedure. On the day of surgery, the patient is instructed to take their usual medications with the exception of insulin, hypoglycemic agents, non-steroidal anti-inflammatory drugs, aspirin, and anticoagulants [21].

The importance of early ambulation needs to be reinforced during the preoperative and in the immediate postoperative period. Patients undergoing bariatric surgical procedures are at greater risk for venous thromboembolism. Mechanical methods (ie, sequential or intermittent pneumatic compression devices) and anticoagulant strategies should be used to prevent the development of deep vein thrombosis and pulmonary embolism [8].

Prophylactic antibiotics are generally recommended to prevent or minimize the risk of surgical site infection [18]. Obesity increases the patient's risk of developing postoperative wound infection. Patients undergoing laparoscopic procedures are

---

Box 3. Preoperative nursing care recommendations

Preoperative nursing care includes:
- Comprehensive admission assessment
- Identification of the patient's support system
- Education of the patient and family about the surgery and postoperative care
- Ensuring a safe physical environment
- Protecting privacy
- Providing size-appropriate equipment and supplies
- Helping the patient with activities of daily living
- Assessment of vital signs, laboratory data, paperwork completion

---

(*Data from* Mulligan A, Young LS, Randall S, et al. Best practices for perioperative nursing care for weight loss surgery patients. Obes Res 2005;13:267–73.)

---

at generally less risk of infection than patients who have open procedures.

Patients may be anxious about the surgical procedure, the anesthesia, and the outcomes of the weight-loss surgery. Preoperative nurses can provide emotional care of the patient, answer questions, and comfort the patient and family before the procedure. Family presence may help the patient relax. Anxiolytics medications may also be needed to help calm the patient (Box 4) [26].

Final preparation

The day of surgery finally arrives. The patient who has actively and willingly participated in preparation for the weight-loss surgery during the extensive preoperative process should be ready and eager to complete the surgical procedure. If the multidisciplinary team of physicians, nurses, physician assistants, dieticians, psychologists, and other support personnel has coordinated the perioperative process and communicated with all involved in the patient's care, the process should be smooth and uncomplicated. The patient's care needs have been met and the patient is ready for

---

**Box 4. Preoperative nursing care:
day of surgery**

Nursing assessment and care on the
day of surgery includes:
• Preventing intraoperative injury: focus
  on special factors that affect
  positioning, physical limitations,
  skin condition
• Sizing of antiembolic stockings and
  sequential compression devices
• Obtaining appropriately sized
  equipment and beds or stretchers
  to facilitate intraoperative and
  postoperative care
• Explaining invasive lines, catheters,
  drains, and analgesic devices
• Education and support of patient
  and family or companions

(*Data from* Mulligan A, Young LS, Randall S,
et al. Best practices for perioperative nursing
care for weight loss surgery patients. Obes
Res 2005;13:267–73.)

---

the surgical experience that will change his or her
life dramatically.

References

[1] Centers for Disease Control and Prevention. Over-
    weight and obesity. Available at: http://www.cdc.
    gov/nccdphp/dnpa/obesity/. Accessed November 21,
    2005.
[2] National Institutes of Health. Clinical guidelines on
    the identification, evaluation, and treatment of over-
    weight and obesity in adults: the evidence report.
    Available at: http://www.nhlbi.nih.gov/guidelines/
    obesity/ob_gdlns.pdf. Accessed November 21, 2005.
[3] Choban PS, Jackson B, Poplawski S, et al. Bariatric
    surgery for morbid obesity: why, who, when, how,
    where, and then what? Cleve Clin J Med 2002;69:
    897–903.
[4] Buchwald H. Overview of bariatric surgery. J Am
    Coll Surg 2002;194:367–75.
[5] Brolin RE. Gastric bypass. Surg Clin North Am
    2001;81:1077–95.
[6] Buchwald H. Consensus conference statement: bari-
    atric surgery for morbid obesity. Health implications
    for patients, health professionals, and third-party
    payers. J Am Coll Surg 2005;200:593–604.
[7] Inderberg CM. The comprehensive care of the bari-
    atric patient: learning the essentials of a successful
    bariatric program. Gundersen Lutheran Medical
    Journal 2004;3:43–50.
[8] Lehman Center Weight Loss Surgery Expert Panel.
    Commonwealth of Massachusetts Betsy Lehman
    Center for Patient Safety and Medical Error Reduc-
    tion Expert Panel on Weight Loss Surgery executive
    report–August 4, 2004. Obes Res 2005;13:205–26.
[9] Saltzman E, Anderson W, Apovian CM, et al. Crite-
    ria for patient selection and multidisciplinary evalu-
    ation and treatment of the weight loss surgery
    patient. Obes Res 2005;13:234–43.
[10] Villagra VG. A primer on bariatric surgery: treat-
    ment of last resort for morbid obesity. Dis Manage
    2004;7(Suppl 1):S23–30.
[11] Nagle AP, Prystowsky JB. Surgical management of
    obesity. Clin Obstet Gynecol 2004;47:928–41.
[12] Garza SF. Bariatric weight loss surgery: patient ed-
    ucation, preparation, and follow-up. Critical Care
    Nursing Quarterly 2003;26:101–4.
[13] Schumann R, Jones SB, Ortiz VE, et al. Best practice
    recommendations for anesthetic perioperative care
    and pain management in weight loss surgery. Obes
    Res 2005;13:254–66.
[14] American Society of Anesthesiologists Task Force
    on Preanesthesia Evaluation. Practice Advisory for
    preanesthesia evaluation: a report by the Ameri-
    can Society of Anesthesiologists Task Force on
    Preanesthesia Evaluation. Anesthesiology 2002;96:
    485–96.
[15] LeMont D, Moore MK, Parish MS, et al. Sugges-
    tions for the pre-surgical psychological assessment
    of bariatric surgery candidates. Available at: http://
    www.asbs.org/html/pdf/PsychPreSurgicalAssessment.
    pdf. Accessed November 21, 2005.
[16] Conte ATH. Critical care pathways for the bariatric
    patient with obstructive sleep apnea. ASCCA Inter-
    change 2004;16:8–9.
[17] Rennotte MT, Baele P, Aubert G, et al. Nasal con-
    tinuous positive airway pressure in the perioperative
    management of patients with obstructive sleep ap-
    nea submitted to surgery. Chest 1995;107:367–74.
[18] Abir F, Bell R. Assessment and management of the
    obese patient. Crit Care Med 2004;32(Suppl. 4):S87–91.
[19] Eagle KA, Berger PB, Calkins H, et al. ACC/AHA
    Guideline update for perioperative cardiovascular
    evaluation for noncardiac surgery–executive sum-
    mary: a report of the American College of Cardiol-
    ogy/American Heart Association Task Force on
    Practice Guidelines (committee to update the 1996
    guidelines on perioperative cardiovascular evalua-
    tion for noncardiac surgery). Anesth Analg 2002;
    94:1052–64.
[20] Moores LK. Smoking and postoperative pulmonary
    complications: an evidence-based review of the re-
    cent literature. Clin Chest Med 2000;21:139–46.
[21] Ogunnaike BO, Jones SB, Jones DB, et al. Anes-
    thetic considerations for bariatric surgery. Anesth
    Analg 2002;95:1793–805.
[22] Breenhaar B, vandenBorne HW, Mullen PD. In-
    adequacies of surgical patient education. Patient
    Education and Counseling 1996;28:31–44.

[23] Lithner M, Zilling T. Pre- and postoperative information needs. Patient Educ Couns 2000;40: 29–37.

[24] Garretson S. Benefits of pre-operative information programmes. Nurs Stand 2004;18:33–7.

[25] American Society of Anesthesiologists. Practice guidelines for the perioperative management of patients with obstructive sleep apnea. Available at: http://www.asahq.org/publicationsAndServices/sleepapnea103105.pdf. Accessed November 25, 2005.

[26] Mulligan A, Young LS, Randall S, et al. Best practices for perioperative nursing care for weight loss surgery patients. Obes Res 2005;13:267–73.

ELSEVIER
SAUNDERS

Perioperative Nursing Clinics 1 (2006) 55–59

PERIOPERATIVE
NURSING
CLINICS

Care of the Obese Patient in the ICU

Lynn Randall, RN, BSN, MBA-HCM*

US Surgical, Norwalk, CT, USA

The growing number of obese patients in critical care units requires special needs and considerations that differ from the normal-weighted patient. The belief is that the obese patient has a stronger body mass, thereby requiring less care. It is also believed that these patients are able to withstand much more pain and insult to the body chemistry because of their size. This could not be further from the truth. Overweight or obese patients are much more fragile than patients of normal weight. Their stability is variable and often these patients cannot take the stress that a critical illness doles out. The more weight a patient carries, the less reserve they have to withstand a major illness.

This article makes nurses aware of the special needs of the obese patient. Reviewed are the cardiovascular, respiratory, and other systems that make the obese patient high risk. Also examined is bariatric surgery, to increase awareness of changes that occur with bariatric surgical procedures and adapt nursing care to accommodate these changes.

Types of bariatric procedures

Biliopancreatic diversion with duodenal switch

Bariatric surgery became prominent in the 1960s. One of the procedures that pioneered bariatric surgery is still being used today, called the biliopancreatic diversion with duodenal switch procedure. In the procedure, a modified gastrectomy is performed along with a bypass of a large portion of the small intestine. This procedure mainly produces a decrease in the absorption of calories and nutrients, most especially fats, thereby causing weight loss. These patients must be monitored carefully for nutritional deficits to ensure that proper calories, vitamins, and minerals are consumed to adjust for the change in absorption (Fig. 1).

Adjustable banded gastroplasty

The adjustable banded gastroplasty is performed by placing a polymeric silicone ring around the fundus of the stomach causing a pseudopouch. Patients feel fuller faster and tend to eat less, causing a reduction in caloric intake. Many patients have been opting for this procedure because it produces the minimal amount of change to the digestive tract (Fig. 2).

Roux-en-Y procedure

The third type of procedure, Roux-en-Y, is considered the gold standard by the American Society of Bariatric Surgeons. A small pouch of approximately 15 to 20 mL (ie, the size of a thumb) is created from the stomach. The small intestine is then divided and reattached to the pouch. The other end is attached again to the small intestine. This procedure provides two methods of weight control. First, it is a restrictive procedure because of the size of the pouch. Decreasing the size of the stomach causes a decreased intake of food.

The Roux-en-Y is also a malabsorptive procedure in that it causes a decrease in absorption of calories because of the bypass of most of the small intestine. The combination of both the restrictive and malabsorptive properties plays an important role in the weight loss of the patient (Fig. 3).

When caring for these patients, nurses must be aware of the malabsorption that takes place

* 3180 Shoreline Drive, Clearwater, FL 33750.
E-mail address: Earlynn.randall@tycohealthcare.com

1556-7931/06/$ - see front matter © 2006 Elsevier Inc. All rights reserved.
doi:10.1016/j.cpen.2005.12.005

periopnursing.theclinics.com

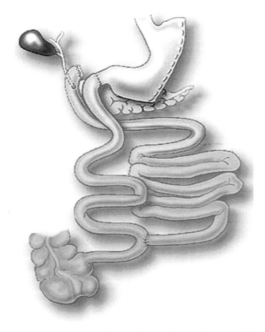

Fig. 1. Biliopancreatic diversion with duodenal switch. (Courtesy of US Surgical, Norwalk, CT; with permission.)

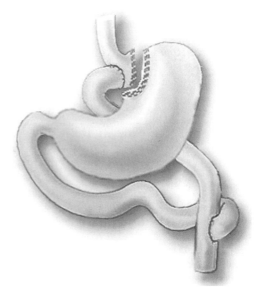

Fig. 3. Roux-en-Y procedure. (Courtesy of US Surgical, Norwalk, CT; with permission.)

following either the Roux-en-Y or duodenal switch procedures. Medication absorption can vary considerably depending on the type of medication and the amount of small bowel that has been bypassed. Nutritional absorption changes that occur with these procedures also require intervention.

Complications following gastric bypass procedures

Two complications that can occur following gastric bypass procedures are anastomotic and thromboembolic. These complications can result in patients returning to surgery, increased length of stay, and even death.

Leaks occur at the gastrojejunostomy anastomosis. A leak can occur within the first 7 to 10 days following surgery. It can be difficult to diagnose because abdominal pain is not always easy to assess; it is often confused with incisional or postsurgical pain. The primary indicator that a postoperative gastric bypass patient may be developing a leak is a tachycardia of 120 or greater [1]. Other signs include fever; back, left shoulder, or abdominal pain; abdominal distention; shortness of breath; and decreased urinary output. If the leak is small, the surgeon may decide to keep the patient on a nothing-by-mouth basis to allow the site to heal on its own. Surgeons

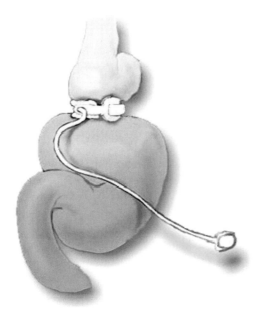

Fig. 2. Adjustable banded gastroplasty. (Courtesy of US Surgical, Norwalk, CT; with permission.)

often prefer to take the patient directly back to surgery to repair the leaking area.

Another complication that can be seen following gastric bypass surgery is deep vein thrombosis (DVT) resulting in pulmonary embolism (PE). Although leaks tend to be more common, a PE results in a patient's death much faster than a leak. It is better to try to prevent than to try to heal a PE [2]. The use of anticoagulation along with sequential compression devices helps in decreasing the risk of a DVT or PE [3].

The obese patient in the ICU

Although the previously listed complications may bring a patient to the ICU for a short stay, many patients who have a body mass index of greater than 40 are admitted to the ICU following other procedures. These patients present a greater risk for complications because of their health status. Because of the changes that occur with body mass index of greater than 40, the special needs of all obese patients must be examined.

Cardiovascular and circulatory status

Obese patients have higher stress on their cardiovascular system. The heart must pump harder to provide adequate perfusion throughout the body. Many of these patients have a higher cardiac output than normal because of the increased stress placed on the heart [4]. This higher cardiac output allows for adequate perfusion throughout the body and should not be decreased rapidly because it can decrease perfusion. The obese patient's body compensates for the higher cardiac output and needs to maintain this to ensure proper blood supply to all tissues.

Obese patients have a higher incidence of congestive heart failure and often have pulmonary hypertension. The pulmonary hypertension is caused by increased preload exacerbated by adipose tissue. This can also lead to right ventricular dysfunction and left ventricular hypertrophy. In a long-term follow-up study to the Framingham Heart Study [5], obese patients have double the risk of heart failure when compared with patients of normal weight.

Interventions include monitoring fluids, pulmonary artery pressures, cardiac output and indexes, and assessing for signs of congestive heart failure and overload. Fluids should be administered judiciously with careful consideration to prevent overload. Because of the high

risk for DVT, sequential compression devices should be applied preoperative and anticoagulant therapy of continuous low-dose intravenous heparin is administered to decrease the risk for DVT development [6].

Respiratory status

Gas exchange in the obese patient poses challenges for the critical care team. During normal inspiration, air enters the lungs pushing the diaphragm down along with the abdominal contents. In the obese patient, however, abdominal fat prevents full expansion of the diaphragm, reducing functional residual capacity. Expansion and gas exchange within the lungs is limited. This chronic limitation can lead to pulmonary shunting and decreased oxygenation. The result is increased difficulty breathing [7].

Sleep apnea is also a known comorbidity of obesity. This chronic condition can lead to prolonged hypoxemia, which in turn can lead to polycythemia in conjunction with pulmonary hypertension. In patients needing ventilatory support, a noninvasive system for oxygen support should be considered if warranted by the patient's condition.

For those patients who require mechanical ventilation, the common practice is to "rest" the lungs for the first 24 to 48 hours. The key is to prevent respiratory muscle fatigue [8]. When initiating mechanical ventilation, it is recommended that tidal volumes be calculated based on the patient's ideal body weight (IBW) rather than the patient's actual body weight (ABW) [9]. Using ABW for tidal volume can cause higher airway pressures and alveolar distention. A study conducted at the University Hospital Lausanne in Switzerland noted that there was a decrease in atelectasis in obese patients immediately after induction of anesthesia if positive end-expiratory pressure was used during induction [10].

The goal when positioning the obese patient is to increase respiratory exchange and improve overall cardiovascular status. It is recommended that the patient be placed in reverse Trendelenburg's position with the head of the bed elevated. This creates a downward movement of abdominal contents, allowing for maximum expansion of the diaphragm.

Renal status

One of the significant comorbidities of obesity is hypertension. Prolonged hypertension can cause renal insufficiency. The postoperative bariatric patient has a negative fluid balance along with malabsorption properties associated with the surgery. Fluid administration can help to maintain fluid balance and preserve glomerular filtration rates.

In the obese patient who has not had bariatric surgery, maintaining fluid balance is crucial. Careful administration of fluids is essential to prevent overload and pulmonary edema.

Another consideration is that of rhabdomyolysis (RML). This is a clinical and biochemical syndrome caused by skeletal muscle necrosis that results in extravasation of toxic intracellular contents from the myocytes into the circulatory system. It is a potentially fatal complication of bariatric surgery. Obese patients are more likely to develop RML than patients of normal weight. The signs of RML are muscle pain and swelling, increased total creatine kinase, narrowed blood urea nitrogen/creatinine ratio, and metabolic acidosis. The RML indicator is the increased creatine kinase. This is considered the rhabdo marker [11]. If this condition is not treated with fluids to flush out the myoglobin, the patient can develop renal failure [12]. Also, potassium can bind with calcium causing a shift in blood levels. One should watch for this in laboratory values [13].

One of the issues with RML is that of acidosis. It has been shown that furosemide can increase the acidosis in a patient. It is recommended to use bumetanide to decrease the acidic nature within the patient [14].

Pharmacology

Research to determine pharmacologic dosages appropriate for obese patients still needs to be completed. The current theory is that dosing should be based on the adjusted body weight (please see computation listed below) rather than the ABW. In patients with chronic illness, there may be decreased protein stores associated with malnourishment. A decrease in protein stores decreases the binding capacity of many medications.

Such medications as anxiolytics, analgesics, and antidepressants are taken up by the adipose tissue and released slowly. Caution must be taken to prevent overdosing bariatric patients with these medications. The medications also might not take full effect as quickly as they would in a normal-weight patient. The patient's response to medications must be assessed to determine if the expected responses are met.

Because of the increased fat to muscle ratio, medication uptake may vary considerably. Because muscle tissue holds more water than fat, medications with hydrophilic distribution may not be distributed to all adipose tissue. Antimicrobials are one drug category that may be affected. To maximize the benefits, the serum concentration of the medication must be monitored. Lipophilic drugs can also cause a prolonged effect even after they are discontinued because of the distribution within the adipose tissue. Some such drugs are fentanyl, propofol, diazepam, and lorazepam [13].

Nutrition

There is a misconception that obese patients are well nourished; this is a fallacy. Many obese patients, especially those with chronic illness, present with varying levels of malnourishment. Obese patients are not able to use fat stores efficiently for energy but instead rely on protein for their energy source, which can result in muscle wasting and decrease healing.

Oral nutritional support should begin as soon as respiratory and cardiovascular stability are achieved. There is discussion in the literature as to the correct caloric intake for the obese patient. Using ABW may actually increase caloric intake past the caloric needs of the patient and cause overload, thereby stressing the cardiovascular and respiratory systems. It has also been suggested, however, that using the IBW may not deliver the necessary calories for the obese patient. The current recommendation is to use adjusted body weight: $(AdjBW = 0.25[ABW-IBW] + IBW)$ [13,15].

Skin breakdown

Skin breakdown is a great concern because with the obese patient it can occur quite rapidly. Multiple skin folds, adipose tissue, and body composition add to the increased risk for decubiti. The time that the patient is on the operating room bed because of the length of procedure and time in one position can attribute to skin breakdown. Fatty tissue has inadequate blood supply. If an obese patient develops a decubitus, it is more difficult to heal. Also, protein stores are often depleted especially in a postoperative gastric bypass patient. This causes a delay in the healing process.

The best advice is to avoid skin breakdown at all costs. The skin must be assessed several times during the day to be sure pressure points are well supported. Maintain clean and dry skin. Do not use powders or thick ointments because they can build up over time making them a prime breeding ground for bacteria.

Beds must be large enough to accommodate the patient's size. Side rails should not cause any pressure points on the patient. Turn the patient every 2 hours and adequately support extremities [16].

Mobility of the obese patient should begin as soon as the patient is stable. Mobility increases perfusion, increases gas exchange, and decreases the risk of DVT. There are many devices on the market today to assist with movement of the critically ill obese patient to minimize the possibility of decubiti formation. The most tried and true intervention to reduce decubiti formation is turning the patient every 2 hours, ensuring that pressure points are supported. As soon as able, patients should sit in a chair and participate in as many activities as tolerated.

Summary

The increase in obesity has been dramatic over the past several years. Caregivers must be prepared to care for these patients with their special needs. The comorbidities associated with obesity can put patients at a severe disadvantage when faced with a critical illness. It is the responsibility of health care workers to ensure proper care of these individuals by knowing the pathophysiology of the obese patient.

Obese patients have distinct changes in their physiology. Cardiac and respiratory systems do not have the ability to withstand dramatic changes, thereby making patients at higher risk for complications. When caring for these individuals, one must be aware of the bariatric-specific needs and address them to achieve the optimal outcome.

References

[1] Tarnoff M. Auto suture bariatric training course. In: Bariatric surgery- historical perspectives: laparoscopic gastric bypass- recognition and management of complications. Philadelphia: WB Saunders; 2003.

[2] Price BL. ASBS allied health essentials course: postoperative complications following bariatric surgery. Aliso Viejo (CA): AACN Critical Care Journals; 2003.

[3] Hess DS, Hess DW. Biliopancreatic diversion with a duodenal switch. Obes Surg 1998;8:267–82.

[4] Karason K, Wallentin I, Larsson B, et al. Effects of obesity and weight loss on cardiac function and valvular performance. Obes Res 1998;6:422–9.

[5] Kenchaiah S, Evans JC, Levy D, et al. Obesity and the risk of heart failure. N Engl J Med 2002;347:305–13.

[6] Quebbemann B, Akhondzadeh M, Dallal R. Continuous intravenous heparin infusion prevents perioperative thromboembolic events in bariatric patients. Obes Surg 2005;15:1221–4.

[7] Battistella FD. Ventilation in the trauma and surgical patient. Crit Care Clin 1998;4:731–42.

[8] Nowbar S, Burkhart KM, Gonzalez R, et al. Obesity association hypoventilation in hospitalized patients: prevalence, effects and outcome. Denver (CO): University of Colorado Health Sciences; 2002.

[9] Marik P, Varon J. The obese patient in the ICU. Chest 1998;113:492–8.

[10] Coussa M, Proiettia S, Schnyder P, et al. Prevention of atelectasis formation during the induction of general anesthesia in morbidly obese patients. Anesth Analg 2004;98:1491–5.

[11] Khourana RN, Baudendistal TE, Morgan EF, et al. Postoperative rhabdomyolysis following laparoscopic gastric bypass in the morbidly obese. Arch Surg 2004;139:73–6.

[12] Cridldle LM. Rhabdomyolysis, pathophysiology, recognition and management. Critical Care Nurse 2003;23:14–30.

[13] Charlebois D, Wilmoth D. Critical care of patients with obesity. Critical Care Nurse 2004;24:19–27.

[14] Collier B, Goreja MA, Duke BE III. Postoperative rhabdomyolysis with bariatric surgery. Obes Surg 2003;6:941–3.

[15] Wurtz R, Itokazu G, Rodvold K. Antimicrobial dosing in obese patients. Clin Infect Dis 1997;25:112–8.

[16] Ahrens T, Kollef M, Stewart J, et al. Effect of kinetic therapy on pulmonary complications. Am J Crit Care 2004;13:376–83.

ELSEVIER
SAUNDERS

Perioperative Nursing Clinics 1 (2006) 61–65

PERIOPERATIVE
NURSING
CLINICS

Truth Telling: An Adjunct to Bariatric Care

Rita C. Scheidt, RNC, BSN

*Department of Continuing Education and Staff Development, MedCentral Health System,
335 Glessner Avenue, Mansfield, OH 44903, USA*

Bariatric "surgery is currently the most effective treatment for morbid obesity resulting in significant weight loss and accompanying health improvements" [1]. This statement, found on the American Obesity Association's web site, presents positive outcomes of surgical intervention to provide hope to patients who are searching for an end to what is often a lifelong struggle with morbid obesity. The Agency for Health Care Research and Quality in a press release states, "The number of Americans having weight-loss surgery more than quadrupled between 1998 and 2002—from 13,386 to 71,733…" [2]. The statistical calculations of their study predict that by 2010 the number of people who are medically eligible for weight loss surgery will reach 475,000 [2].

This trend has profound implications for health care in a variety of settings. In physician offices, clinics, and hospitals, especially facilities where bariatric care is provided, the need for education, a commitment to excellence, attention to epidemiologic trends, and a dedication to uncompromising attentiveness to patient needs and health status are critical. Physicians and nurses are in a unique position to contribute to the patient's well-being by being generous with the knowledge they have and thereby increasing the potential for health care decisions that prevent devastating results. The patient has the obligation and duty to take an active role in learning, asking questions, and using every opportunity to ferret out the information that leads to the best health care decision for them. In this way, health care provider and patient join forces in making the decisions and choices that lead to health and wholeness based on an accurate interpretation of facts and figures. Patients who struggle with obesity have a need for details that help them unravel the enormous volume of data available. The reality providers must recognize is that patients have access to sources of information unavailable in the not too distant past. The World Wide Web is a repository of both accurate and inaccurate health care information. One must also consider the vulnerability of patients who are weary of the stressors, strain, and ill health that often accompany obesity. Considering the high number of patients who seek weight loss surgery, it is likely that many do so out of desperation. Nurses and physicians need to recognize how easily some patients may choose surgery over alternative routes to a higher level of fitness and better health. Bariatric surgery is, for a select number of patients, the only hope for weight reduction. Providers have an obligation to tell patients the truth, without involvement in the distortions promoted by the dearth of sensationalism and misinformation available. For some, despite the best care and preoperative preparation, weight loss surgery is the beginning of a progressive decline in health leading to dire consequences, serious complications, or death. Indeed, for some it begins a journey best not begun.

The US Department of Health and Human Services, the Department of Disease Prevention and Public Health, in partnership with other federal agencies, state and territorial health departments, businesses, and numerous other agencies have developed and established a compilation of objectives that contribute to disease prevention and health promotion. This national initiative is called Healthy People 2010 [3]. These

E-mail address: jscheidt@neo.rr.com

objectives, developed by scientists within government agencies and the private sector, specify two primary goals: increase quality and years of healthy life, and eliminate health disparities. To move the nation toward these goals leading health indicators were named, and these are used to measure the health of the nation over the first 10 years of this century [3]. In a brochure explaining this initiative, overweight-obesity is identified as one of several disease entities of concern [4]. The numbers of people who qualify for bariatric surgery in 2010, if accurate, suggest that reaching these hopeful and extraordinary goals is far from ensured.

A recent issue of the *Journal of the American Medical Association* included several articles about some aspect of bariatric surgery. One article in particular, "Early mortality among Medicare beneficiaries undergoing bariatric surgical procedures," triggered multiple reports in the media that announced the results of studies that reveal disturbing facts about the consequences of surgical intervention for weight reduction [5]. The details of these studies have been widely reported and focus on the risks, negative outcomes, and complications following bariatric surgery. Although many of these reports about the research findings restricted reporting to the facts, the tone embodied by most was one of alarm.

The titles and opening statements in some of these reports highlight the darker side of bariatric surgery, sounding a clarion call toward a more balanced representation of the benefits and complications of surgery for morbid obesity. A report on CBS News, "Study: obesity surgery risky," begins with the sentence, "A new study shows that the chances of dying within a year after obesity surgery are higher that previously thought, even among people in their 30s and 40s" [6]. Dr. David Flum of the University of Washington, a bariatric surgeon, states, "The risk of death is much higher than has been reported...It's a reality check for those patients who are considering these surgeries." His words are sobering and alarming in light of the popularization of weight loss surgery. The article stated that Medicare patients may be sicker, but that negative complications have decreased as surgeons' expertise increased [6]. Such conclusions are of little comfort to patients having to contend with leaks, hernias, vitamin deficiencies, hair loss, feeding tubes, and second or even third surgeries. After reading patient accounts of personal experiences with complications, one is startled by the contrast between such devastating results and testimonials that convey elation and joy at having dropped massive amounts of weight and bask in the glory of "feeling normal for the first time in their lives."

"Gastric bypass: let the morbidly obese beware" appeared on MedPage Today in a review about a news article from Forbes, NBC, Newsletter. The article warns, "Gastric bypass is on the rise, and so are the rates of hospitalizations and early postoperative deaths related to complications." Although the article also points out that bariatric surgery is appropriate for select patients and by select surgeons "experience and technique count" [7].

Other citations include "Study: obesity surgery carries hidden risks" at USAToday.com [8], and "Studies point to risks of last-resort operation" [9] from the Houston Chronicle's on-line issue. A UW Medicine, University of Washington, news release announced, "Bariatric surgery deaths higher for older Medicare patients" [10]. From rxpgnews comes the news summary, "Gastric bypass surgery patients have double the rate of hospitalizations" [11]. The web search list goes on, one article after another, each declaring that the positive aspects of bariatric surgery have eclipsed the negative. It may indicate, at best, that patients and health care providers have not had a comprehensive valuation of the benefits and risks associated with this surgery. At worst, these reports imply that the negative consequences of weight loss surgery, although known, have not been fully explained to patients. Both of these assumptions are worth considering. Health care providers have an opportunity to make use of this research and use it to inform and guide their practice. The potential for increased patient safety and improved outcomes is irrefutable.

In an interview, a patient shared her personal experience with bariatric surgery. When asked at 3.5 weeks postoperative if she was glad of her decision for bariatric surgery, she said, "The jury is still out." She reported no serious complications and was pleased with her weight loss and reduction of knee and back pain. She was eating a wide variety of foods, but was finding it difficult to consume the food she needed to maintain good nutrition. She had researched and educated herself. She experienced doubt and at one point believed that "the bariatric surgery business was a racket." She considered the risks, discussed all aspects of what this surgery would mean, not only for her personal well-being, but her relationships to spouse and family. She even believed that she could lose the weight without it, but ultimately she made the decision to have surgery because she did not believe that she could keep it off. After deciding, she had to wait 6 months before she could actually schedule her surgery. Today she feels stronger, but has both good and bad days. When asked if she would do it again, she replied, "The jury is still out." She is losing her hair.

This patient had a friend who also had bariatric surgery, had a leak, a hernia, several hospital admissions, and even had a feeding tube for a while. She had lost 150 pounds. Would she do it again? She said, "Yes, in a heartbeat!" One can only ask, why? "Because," she said, "I feel so good about myself now." Reflecting on this experience, one can only speculate about the extent of the pain she endured before surgery (it must have been great), and then the daring that enabled her to endure such a degree of post-operative suffering and still say, "Yes, I would do it again, in a heartbeat."

Questions must be asked, and discussions are needed, for care providers to deliver the kind of care that endeavors to reach the best decision for the patient, even if it means denying surgical intervention. Does the patient education provided thoroughly disclose the risk of all potential complications? Does the informed consent instruct the patient about what may happen, in a way that is all-inclusive of potentialities? Is the necessity of absolute compliance, for positive results, spelled out in the details? Are the long-term changes in eating, activity, and lifestyle cited? For each patient, what may contribute to the choice to have surgery? What factors should tip the scales and result in no procedure at all, but rather provide encouragement for an alternative route to weight loss?

What role does the physician or other health care provider have in the decision-making process? Even if the surgery is done because of serious comorbidities, what contribution does the provider make that escorts the patient to or away from the operating room table? A number of these questions have concrete answers. Some require a willingness to enter into a dialog that is brutally honest, yet laced with a heavy dose of compassion and empathy.

Critical thinking that uses the tools of ethical decision making may lead to less and not more bariatric surgery procedures. The US Department of Human Services in a news release in July of 2004 announced a policy change in Medicare's coverage for obesity treatment. Tommy G. Thompson, Health and Human Services Secretary, indicated that Medicare would remove barriers to coverage for interventions for obesity "if scientific and medical evidence demonstrate their effectiveness in improving Medicare beneficiaries' health outcomes" [12]. It will be interesting to see how reports impact pubic policy for recipients of Medicare coverage. In light of recent reporting, the US Department of Human Service on Healthfinder: Health Highlights on May 27, 2005, indicates that, "Due to risks incurred as a result of gastric bypass some insurance companies are dropping coverage" [13]. The logical consequence of this phenomenon is that people who want this surgery may not be able to have it.

The efforts to support a patient's choice for surgery include those used by Gant [14], who provides services for a facility in Texas and administers various psychologic tools to measure the probability of postprocedure compliance. This effort to contribute to positive patient outcomes is evidence of teamwork in bariatric treatment modalities.

Semuels [15] writes about a woman who discovered post–bariatric surgery that her depression did not subside. Although initially she was ecstatic about her weight loss, she concluded that gastric bypass "is not the cure-all that some expect it to be." She found that it was not the "silver bullet" she had hoped. In the same article, in the time frame between 2004 and 2005, three patients committed suicide, all of them post–bariatric surgery. A forensic neuropathologist with the coroner's office acknowledged that "The risk of suicide does not go down with body weight. The surgery does not cure depressive illness" [15]. Providers stress that depression is not necessarily a reason not to do the surgery; major depressive illness is a condition that should be addressed and treated before surgery. It is a common practice for patients to undergo psychologic screening and evaluation before the final decision to go ahead with bariatric surgery [15]. Some comprehensive programs take a holistic approach and pay careful attention to presurgery screening and postoperative follow-up.

Tao and Glazer [16], in the Online Journal of Issues in Nursing, discuss "Obesity: from a health issue to a political and policy issue." They declare two ways in which obesity becomes an item included on the political agenda: the increasingly higher cost associated with obesity, perceived to be at an unacceptable level, motivates legislators to address issues that contribute to the increase;

and obesity, like smoking (addiction), perceived by many to be a matter of personal choice, has become a public health matter with significant regulation, and "obesity as a political issue has surpassed obesity as a health issue." This resulted in a national "War on Obesity."

Stakeholders identified in the article are "the government, the food industry, health care providers, employers, and the middle class." Each aspires to influence public policy. For example: changes in Medicare and Medicaid benefits result in fluctuations in the direction and focus of government spending. It is likely that some issues, depending on the stakeholders involved, may find their way into a legislator's efforts for re-election [16].

Regarding the food industry, policy changes may have both a positive and negative effect depending on point of view. The food industry has sought to pass laws that ensure protection from liability, by altering suggested national dietary guidelines, or recommendations for increased activity levels. The focus promoted by nutritionists is different. Their focus is primarily one of advocacy, such as promoting legislation to detoxify the food environment [16].

The benefits sought by health care providers are more complex in that they include diagnosis, prevention, and treatment. Pressure from this sector may produce a variety of policies that may have to do with health promotion, screenings, issues of advocacy, and funding for research. The change in how the IRS has modified their stand on deductions for obesity treatment, may have led to an improvement in insurance coverage. This has led to an increase in demand for obesity treatment and a decrease in uncompensated care [16].

Because of this war on obesity and the escalating cost of treatment modalities, employers and the public are concerned about the projected tax burden and diminishing profits. Furthermore, this tax burden may then drive the cost of insurance premiums to a level that is likely to be passed on to the consumer resulting in a reduction in wages. These are a few of the specifics that consign obesity to the center stage of public policy and political maneuvering [16].

Tao and Glazer [16] foster the notion that nurses are not perceived as stakeholders, and so are in a position to influence the political process and advocate for access to safe health care. Nurses who are highly committed to the role of patient advocate can choose to lobby for initiatives that have a positive influence on the health of not only individuals, but in the promotion of a healthy society and communities that support positive, healthy lifestyles.

What can individual health care providers do beyond asking the right questions? There are four precepts that may be of value to providers, physicians, nurses, dieticians, physical trainers, counselors, or anyone who takes part in the care given bariatric patients. One could extend their application to all opportunities for interaction with all patients seeking health care of any kind. The first is respect. Respect for the person, their values, beliefs, thinking, ideas, choices, and decisions. This respect extends to aspects and characteristics that may be repugnant, offensive, or distasteful. Respect or esteem that maintains a healthy intellectual humility in every interaction with the patient. Recognize that often care providers can learn a great deal from the patient that ultimately deepens and enriches their practice. The second is the intention to maintain an awareness of perspective, especially in assessment, evaluation, and treatment. The caregiver has an obligation to take into account that there is often a multitude of perspectives, and considering this enhances communication and promotes understanding. The third is perseverance, the resolution to exercise tenacity in the pursuit of the most effective approach that guides the patient toward health promotion that may, or may not, include bariatric surgery. Fourth is to use all of these precepts with uncompromising integrity that cultivates a firm and solid foundation for the delivery of consistent and trustworthy medical care.

Obesity is a multifaceted condition. Each patient's experience is distinct and unique to their person. There is no "one size fits all" treatment option that eliminates the changes required that leads to weight loss and ultimate weight control. Weight loss surgery is forced transformation. The surgery imposes a change in eating habits, activity levels, and other alterations in lifestyle. Although success is certain for some, a triumph over a life-long search for health, for others it has the potential for failure. To serve patients well, they are best served by a proactive commitment, by joining forces with them in their quest for the answer that for them is pivotal. Engaging in candid dialog and sharing their journey by telling the truth without sensationalizing the facts makes truth-telling an adjunct to bariatric care.

References

[1] American Obesity Association. Morbid obesity: AOA fact sheet. Available at: http://www.obesity.org/subs/fastfacts/morbidobesity.shtml. Accessed October 15, 2005.

[2] Agency for Healthcare Research and Quality. AHRQ study finds weight-loss surgeries quadrupled in five years. Available at: http://www.ahrq.gov/news/press/pr2005/wtlosspr.htm. Accessed August 22, 2005.

[3] US Department of Health and Human Services. Healthy people 2010. Available at: http://www.healthypeople.gov/About/hpfact.htm. Accessed August 22, 2005.

[4] US Department of Health and Human Services. Steps to a healthier US. Available at: http://www.healthierus.gov/steps/steps_brochure.pdf. Accessed August 22, 2005.

[5] Flum DR, Salem L, Broeckel Elrod J, et al., Early mortality among Medicare beneficiaries undergoing bariatric surgical procedures. Available at: http://jama.ama-assn.org/cgi/reprint/294/15/1903. Accessed October 29, 2005.

[6] CBS News. Study: obesity surgery risky. Available at: http://www.cbsnews.com/stories/2005.10/18/health/printable953870.shtml. Accessed November 5, 2005.

[7] Osterwell N. Gastric bypass: let the morbidly obese beware. Available at: http://medpagetoday.com/tbprint.cfm?bid=1958. Accessed November 5, 2005.

[8] USA Today. Study: obesity surgery carries hidden risks. Available at: http://usatoday.printthis.clickabiity.com/pt/cpt?action=cpt&title=. Accessed November 5, 2005.

[9] Houston Chronical. Studies point to risks of last-resort operation. Available at: http://chron.com.cs/CDA/printsory.mpl/health/3402776. Accessed November 5, 2005.

[10] Sowers P. Bariatric surgery deaths higher for older Medicare patients. Available at: http://uwmedicine.org/Global/NewsAndEvents/PressReleases. Accessed November 5, 2005.

[11] Journal of the American Medical Association. Gastric bypass surgery patients have double the rate of hospitalizations. Available at: http://rxpgnews.com/research/surgery/printer_2666.shtml. Accessed November 5, 2005.

[12] US Department of Health and Human Services. HHS announces revised Medicare obesity coverage policy. Available at: http://hhs.gov/news/pres/20040715.html. Accessed November 5, 2005.

[13] Healthfinder (US Department of Health and Human Services). Risks of weight-loss surgery can impede treatment. Available at: http://www.healthfinder.gov/news/newsstory.asp?docID=525987. Accessed November 5, 2005.

[14] Gant RL. Medical psychology: practical support for differing medical needs. Available at: http://assessments-stage.ncspearson.com/bridginggap/summer2005p1.htm. Accessed November 5, 2005.

[15] Semuels A. Gastric bypass surgery patients often find it's not a cure for depression. Available at: http://www.post-gazette.com/pg/05180/529753.stm. Accessed November 5, 2005.

[16] Tao H, Glazer G. Obesity: from a health issue to a political and policy issue. Available at: http://www.nursingworld.org/ojin/tpclg/leg_15.htm. Accessed July 16, 2005.

ELSEVIER
SAUNDERS

Perioperative Nursing Clinics 1 (2006) 67–71

PERIOPERATIVE
NURSING
CLINICS

Practicing Safe Care of the Bariatric Population

Brenda S. Gregory Crum, RN, MSN, CNOR*

Sandel Medical Industries LLC, Chatsworth, CA, USA

Safe practices are a role that perioperative nurses integrate in every activity of the day. The patient population in areas where operative and invasive procedures occur requires nurses to have a depth of knowledge and ability to care for patients who are compromised and anxious because they are undergoing a procedure. This might result in the patient's inability or lack of willingness to share thoughts, ask questions, or even comprehend what is occurring. The bariatric population offers unique challenges and requires competencies of health care providers to increase awareness and understand potential problems for promoting safe practices.

Bariatric patients might be admitted to an inpatient or outpatient facility, depending on the type of weight loss procedure that is planned. Within surgical settings, risks increase with use of equipment and technology (eg, malfunction, burns, and fires); blood transfusion; communication types and patterns; patient and site identification; medication administration; positioning; and counts. Safety measures appropriate for the perioperative patient population apply with specific considerations for care of obese patients. As a patient's advocate the registered nurses and other health care providers who are caring for patients undergoing bariatric procedures need to recognize the interventions that decrease risk for patients and employees.

Safety measures must be addressed at the time a bariatric program is established so that resources are allocated appropriately for patient and employee educational needs, adequate facilities, and equipment. Successful bariatric programs are multidisciplinary and the team members are responsible for all facets of the patient's care. In addition to understanding the surgical procedure, patient's needs, and adequate preparation, team member and patient communication facilitate safe patient care.

This article reviews high-risk considerations for bariatric care including education, resource allocation, airway and medication management, positioning, and prevention of postoperative complications. The environmental and resource needs in addition to specific problem-prone interventions that must be considered when planning and caring for this patient population are discussed.

Education

Team education for bariatric care includes understanding the surgical procedures in addition to preoperative and postoperative care, patient teaching, physiology, and risk-reduction measures. Challenges occur when educating multidisciplinary health care providers who have not previously focused on the special needs of the obese population because of preconceived opinions and ideas. Time should be allocated for education and sensitivity training to increase awareness of health care providers' understanding of the obese patient's psychosocial needs. The patient is experiencing a surgical procedure and is motivated by the prospect of a lifestyle change that should also improve their health status by improving medical comorbidities (eg, diabetes, cardiovascular disease, sleep apnea, arthritis). Understanding and reinforcing program treatments and supporting requirements for long-term follow-up presents a unified multidisciplinary effort.

Preoperative patient education is believed to be critical to the success of any bariatric surgery. At the time patients are admitted to the health care

* 11105 Castleberry Road, Odessa, FL 34655.
E-mail address: bsgd@aol.com

1556-7931/06/$ - see front matter © 2006 Elsevier Inc. All rights reserved.
doi:10.1016/j.cpen.2005.12.008

setting they have spent considerable time being educated and prepared for one more aspect of their experience. Treatments to reduce risks, such as alveolar hypotension and deep vein thrombosis, are started weeks before admission for the surgical procedure. It is important to understand all of the information shared and requirements to prepare for this procedure to enable health care providers to offer the necessary support and teaching. Consistently reinforcing important information might help patients recall key components of their preoperative education that might otherwise be forgotten, but is necessary for their long-term postoperative success [1].

Most patients undergoing bariatric procedures are the adult population, but because of the prevalence of overweight youth in the United States, and associated comorbidities, there is a growing need for effective weight management interventions for the younger population. In addition to understanding the needs of the adult population, team members should have the knowledge of pediatric and adolescent patient needs to provide the physical and psychosocial support for patients in these populations who might undergo bariatric procedures.

Resource allocation

Determining adequate resources to provide care should be a primary goal to providing safe patient care. Risks associated with inadequate resources might result in employee and patient injury. These resources must be established at the time a bariatric program is established to minimize opportunities for these risks.

The bariatric patient population in addition to the increased weight of all obese patients undergoing procedures mandates that employee staffing is provided adequately to offer necessary assistance. It is expected that the patients will be mobile and ambulate for testing and from preadmission before surgery, yet the size of the patient might warrant transfer in a wheelchair as early as point of entry to the health care facility. During procedures (including endoscopic, radiologic, and surgery) and until the time of discharge, employees are required to assist patients and be responsible for transferring, transporting, positioning, and mobilizing the patient. A consideration for appropriate numbers of personnel to staff all areas where care is provided because of the increased physical demands (eg, transferring,

lifting, and turning) must be paramount as the decisions about resources are made, because employee injury can result in additional hospital costs.

Determining adequate staffing needs is subjective based on the patient's size. The minimal number of persons who routinely complete these activities for patients who are less than 200 lb does not suffice. Recommendations for supine transfer of an awake, noncompromised patient in the supine position (ie, bed to stretcher) is a minimum of three persons and a friction-reducing device for patients greater than 200 lb [2]. The number of persons required for a transfer of the bariatric patient is relative to the size and staffing should be considered to provide adequate patient care. Devices should be used that minimize stress and strain on employees, but the use of devices does not minimize the need for appropriate numbers of personnel. Assistance needed for transfer in wheelchairs, stretchers, and ambulating are activities that must be considered when determining the number of staff who should be available to assist.

Every aspect of the patient's care must be assessed to prepare the health care setting for equipment and supply needs. Waiting room chairs, patient scales, floor-mounted toilets, large-sized gowns, stretchers, wheelchairs, operating room beds, and hospital beds of adequate dimensions without weight limits must be purchased for this patient population [3]. Hydraulic-operated equipment, such as stretchers and lifts, must be available in adequate quantities and accessible. Blood pressure cuffs and sequential compression devices must be of a size that safely fit and function. In addition, facilities may require remodeling to provide doorways and elevators of width that accommodate larger beds, stretchers, and wheelchairs. Patient rooms must be equipped with shower facilities large enough to accommodate an obese person. Safe practices are necessary including keeping hallways clear to allow transfer between locations on a stretcher so that employees are not constantly attempting to move through a maze of equipment or maneuver heavy stretchers around sharp corners.

Patient positioning

Positioning is a critical intervention for any patient's care. The obese patient's physiology and size lend themselves to adverse outcomes if safety factors are not considered. The perioperative nurse must understand the anatomic and physiologic changes associated with the patient's health condition, anesthesia, position, and the operative procedure. Adverse effects on the musculoskeletal, integumentary, nervous, respiratory, and cardiovascular systems must be prevented. The supine position can be challenging simply because of pressure created by the patient's weight.

The preoperative assessment allows the perioperative nurse adequately to plan positioning needs. Age, height, general health status, skin condition, and respiratory, circulatory, and neurologic status require a thorough assessment. Planning activities protect the patient from injury and provide the physiologic support and comfort while allowing for optimal exposure and access to the surgical site. In addition to the correct size and type of equipment, the number of available personnel to transfer and position the patient must be considered to reduce risk of patient and employee injury.

Because the patient's weight is greater than average and they often have secondary health-related conditions (eg, diabetes, circulatory compromise), positioning, supplies, and equipment must be used taking those factors into consideration. When patients are transferred to the operating room bed, the patient's comfort and potential pressure areas are identified and assessed. The patient's weight creates pressure on underlying tissue as gravity presses downward toward the surface of the bed, increasing compromise of tissue, nerves, and even muscle. Rhabdomyolysis has occurred when there is pressure on the muscles for an extended length of time. The specific lengths of time and amount of pressure are not known, but because this can result in a fatal outcome, it is a consideration when positioning [4].

The standard position for patients undergoing bariatric procedures is supine with repositioning during the procedure to reverse Trendelenburg's position. The operating room bed must be of the size that accommodates the patient's weight to prevent injury and allows the team members to reposition using automated equipment. The operating room bed should hold up to 1000 lb with a 600-lb tilt capacity. Attachments are available to provide support for extrawide girth. Draw sheets should be long enough to secure the patient's arms if positioned at the side. A padded footboard with holders prevents the patient from slipping when the bed is placed in reverse Trendelenburg's

position. Arm boards must be wide enough to provide adequate support. If the arms are secured at the side of the patient, it is important to place padding to eliminate nerve damage.

Following anesthesia induction, the respiratory status is maintained, and the patient is assessed head to toe for potential pressure areas or injury and body alignment. The patient is secured across the upper and lower legs with a safety strap. The feet are placed in an anatomically neutral position and secured to the footboard to prevent slippage. Breasts and genitals might require positioning attention to eliminate unnecessary pressure during the procedure.

Postoperative the skin integrity and circulatory status is assessed. As the patient responds following anesthesia the neuromuscular status is also assessed. Attention to positioning needs results in the patient being free from injury related to surgical positioning.

Airway, anesthesia, and pain management

Experience caring for obese patients alters the choices for anesthesia care, pain management, and choices of medications. Comorbidities of obese patients can have the greatest influence on these decisions. The presence of obstructive sleep apnea might require altering anesthetic technique and medications, although there is little evidence to guide this practice. Choices for monitoring blood pressure can differ because of inadequate cuff size, resulting in need for insertion of an arterial line. A central line might be required if there is difficulty inserting peripheral lines.

Pharmacokinetics of obesity is influenced by variations in plasma protein binding, body composition, and blood flow of these patients. Correct dosing has implications for anesthesia delivery and recovery. Obese patients have a greater increase in fat mass as compared with increased lean body mass. Because blood flow to the fat is poor yet blood volume increases with body weight, the increased cardiac output in obese patients results in greater blood flow to viscera. Studies of propofol, opioids, neuromuscular blockers, and volatile anesthetics have been conducted, but plasma concentrations and accumulation of medications requires further study to determine dosing considering total body weight versus ideal body weight [5]. Available studies suggest that dosing according to ideal body weight can be effective with some medications.

Managing the airway is a goal of anesthesia supervision. Decisions to attain this goal might begin preoperative with respiratory treatments. Obesity is associated with reduced expiratory reserve volume, forced vital capacity and forced expiratory volume, functional residual capacity, and maximum voluntary ventilation. Experience with airway management of the obese patient in surgery improves successes because of an understanding of positioning, required equipment, and responses. Induction using a mask airway or an awake intubation is considered following patient assessment to determine needs and limitations. Differing opinions about oxygen delivery exist. Preoxygenation with positive end-expiratory pressure might be considered to reduce the post-intubation arterial oxygenation. The parameters that determine success of using positive end-expiratory pressure have not been established but have shown that advantages exist and the maneuvers should be considered. The goal with oxygen administration is to maintain the respiratory drive to prevent postoperative atelectasis. Postoperative coughing and deep breathing and ambulation should begin as soon as the patient is able to perform.

Sedative and narcotic-based drugs should be administered with caution to prevent exacerbation of symptoms of sleep apnea. Nonsteroidal anti-inflammatory drugs and local anesthetic for incisional infiltration can adjunct the need for large doses of narcotics. Postoperative continuous infusion for pain management has also been used successfully.

Opportunities for research related to medication delivery in obese patients should be completed to determine specific patient care needs and benefits. Anesthesia and pain management and preventive medication therapies result in maintaining the airway, reducing postoperative complications, and relieving postoperative pain.

Postoperative adverse outcomes: deep vein thrombosis and infection

Thromboembolic events, such as deep vein thrombosis, are adverse outcomes associated with bariatric surgery, requiring preventive medication therapy. Studies to determine dosing and peak levels of heparin suggest that low-dose intravenous heparin therapy is associated with low incidence of thromboembolic events and low risk for perioperative hemorrhage [6,7].

As with all surgical procedures, sterile technique is critical. In addition, prophylactic antimicrobial therapy is considered when caring for obese patients because of the preoperative wound classification of "class II/clean contaminated." Adverse outcomes associated with surgical site infections and the potential for occurrence when patients are obese and the alimentary tract is entered warrant use of preoperative antibiotics. They should be ordered and administered so that the bactericidal concentration of the antibiotic is established in serum and tissues by the time the skin is incised [8].

Surgical counts

Retained foreign bodies are estimated to occur at least once a year in health care facilities in which major cases are performed. Obesity is one identified risk for this possibility [9]. Accurate count procedures and standardized counts can significantly reduce the incidence of these events. Measures that can be taken to reduce this risk include (1) executing a careful and thoughtful exploration of the operative site before closure; (2) inspecting instruments in their entirety when setting up the surgical procedure and after use; (3) counting sharps, sponges, and instruments before and following all procedures; (4) using radiograph-detectable items with radiopaque indicators for items that cannot otherwise be detected on radiograph; and (5) not placing nonradiopaque sponges or towels in the wound. This is a specific consideration when patients must return postoperative because of a wound infection that requires packing. Surgical counts have been practiced for years, but in a high-risk situation, such as care of the obese patient, the need to complete an accurate count is a critical intervention. Retained objects is a preventable outcome. Improvements in communication and processes prevent the risk of injury related to retained foreign bodies.

The choice to improve practices

Improving patient safety when caring for obese patients requires the evaluation of risk factors and trends on a national basis. Competency of health care workers providing care for bariatric patients must be assessed, considering the special needs of this patient population. Workplace environments must be improved to accommodate this patient population. The knowledge and responsibilities of perioperative nurses in a highly technical and high-risk environment positions them to demonstrate patient advocacy and make major differences in safety improvements. The commitment to a bariatric program is challenging, but offers opportunities for health care providers to join forces, problem solve, and lead in ways that influence positive outcomes and improvements in the lives of thousands of patients each year.

References

[1] Madan AK, Tichansky DS. Patients postoperatively forget aspects of preoperative patient education. Obes Surg 2005;15 1066–19.

[2] Baptiste A, Kelleher V, Nelson K, et al. Technology resource guide for bariatric patient. Available at: http://www.visn8.med.va.gov/PatientSafetyCenter/resguide/BariTechResGuide.pdf. Accessed January 9, 2006.

[3] Ergonomics Technical Advisory Group. Patient care ergonomics resource guide: safe patient handling and movement. Available at: http://www.visn8.med. va.gov/PatientSafetyCenter/resguide/ErgoGuidePtOne. pdf. Accessed January 9, 2006.

[4] de Menezes Ettinger JE, dos Santos Filho PV, Asaro E, et al. Prevention of rhabdomyolysis in bariatric surgery. Obes Surg 2005;15:874–9.

[5] Passannante AN, Rock P. Anesthetic management of patients with obesity and sleep apnea. Anesthesiol Clin North America 2005;23:479–91.

[6] Prystowsky JB, Morasch MD, Eskandari MK, et al. Prospective analysis of the incidence of deep venous thrombosis in bariatric surgery patients. Surgery 2005; 138:759–63.

[7] Quebbemann B, Akhondzadeh M, Dallal R. Continuous intravenous heparin infusion prevents perioperative thromboembolic events in bariatric surgery patients. Obes Surg 2005;15:1221–4.

[8] Mangram A, Horan TC, Pearson ML, et al. Guideline for prevention of surgical site infection, 1999. Available at: http://www.cdc.gov/ncidod/dhqp/pdf/guidelines/SSI.pdf. Accessed December 5, 2005.

[9] Gwande AA, Srudert DM, Orav TM, et al. Patient safety: risk factors for retained instruments and sponges after surgery. N Engl J Med 2003;348: 229–35.

ELSEVIER
SAUNDERS

Perioperative Nursing Clinics 1 (2006) 73–76

PERIOPERATIVE
NURSING
CLINICS

Index

Note: Page numbers of article titles are in **boldface** type.

periopnursing.theclinics.com

Changing Your Address?

Make sure your subscription changes too! When you notify us of your new address, you can help make our job easier by including an exact copy of your Clinics label number with your old address (see illustration below.) This number identifies you to our computer system and will speed the processing of your address change. Please be sure this label number accompanies your old address and your corrected address—you can send an old Clinics label with your number on it or just copy it exactly and send it to the address listed below.

We appreciate your help in our attempt to give you continuous coverage. Thank you.

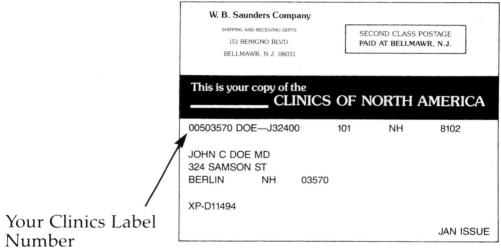

Your Clinics Label Number

Copy it exactly or send your label
along with your address to:
W.B. Saunders Company, Customer Service
Orlando, FL 32887-4800
Call Toll Free 1-800-654-2452

Please allow four to six weeks for delivery of new subscriptions and for processing address changes.